About th

Jacquelynn Luben moved from London on her marriage in 1966, and, in secluded Surrey woodland, she and her husband built the bungalow that has been their home ever since.

After the birth of her son, she suffered two miscarriages before her daughter Amanda was born. When Amanda became a cot death victim at the age of two months, Jacquelynn tried to find out more about cot death or 'Sudden Infant Death Syndrome' and received support and help from The British Guild for Sudden Infant Death Study, later absorbed by The Foundation for the Study of Infant Deaths. This latter organisation was founded in 1971, the same year as Amanda's birth and death, and the author remained in contact with them, carrying out occasional fund raising events on their behalf.

In 1972, Jacquelynn's second daughter was born, and during the same period she started writing about her experience in the form of articles for publication and letters to other bereaved parents. In 1986, her book *Cot Deaths - Coping with Sudden Infant Death Syndrome* was published and has been helpful to parents and health professionals alike.

Since then, she has extended her writing into fiction and poetry, as well as non-fiction. She combines studying for a degree with Surrey University, working on her latest novel and publishing her short stories on line.

By the same author

COT DEATHS - COPING WITH SUDDEN
INFANT DEATH SYNDROME
Published by Bedford Square Press

Fiction on line on the author's website
http://freespace.virginnet.co.uk/luben.glade

THE FRUIT

of the

TREE

Jacquelynn Luben

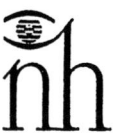

Published in 1992 by Nelson Houtman

Bullswater Common, Pirbright, Woking,

Surrey, GU24 0LY

British Library Cataloguing in Publication Data
Luben, Jacquelynn
  Fruit of the Tree
  I. Title
  920

  ISBN 0-9518894-0-0

Printed and bound in Great Britain by
Antony Rowe Ltd, Chippenham, Wiltshire.

Cover design by MCA

FOREWORD

Jacquelynn Luben's book *The Fruit of the Tree* charts a tragic course which many of us have negotiated and wish would never have to happen to anyone else. Losing a baby and not knowing why is an experience shared by so many of us, and Jacquelynn has had more than her fair share of sadness and difficulties, which she graphically describes in this book.

However, as she demonstrates, the human being is capable of immense strength to bounce back time and time again the face of despair. This book is a tribute to her lost baby, and our crusade to find out why.

ANGELA PERRY (1992)
Appeals Chairman
The Foundation for the Study of Infant Deaths

A Hebrew prayer: Blessed art Thou, oh Lord our God, King
of the Universe, Who createst the fruit of the tree.

Acknowledgements

I should like to thank all those people who have been instrumental in helping *The Fruit of the Tree* on its route to publication.

Professor Bernard Knight, who told me, 'I believe you have a book in you,' and launched me into my literary career; who subsequently was called upon to read my first efforts and advise; Irene Black, who sat and read through with me my first hand-written and untidy manuscript; my mother, Sadie Beaver, and my friend, Miriam Goldsmith, who read the typescript and gave me their comments; Stella Stocker of the Guildford Writers' Workshop, who gave me detailed constructive criticism; my daughter, Karen, who copy-typed the whole manuscript into my word processor, when I could not face another retyping; to Peter Finch, author, poet and former publisher, for reassurance and support. Finally, thanks to my friendly old Imperial 55 typewriter, on whom I typed all my early works, until it was supplanted by new technology.

Contents

After the Lord Mayor's Show

I opened the heavy front door. Outside, the main road was grey with rain and I hesitated in the doorway. My parents were upstairs, still presumably directing operations.

A middle-aged Jewish couple were walking along the pavement. The woman glanced in my direction, then stopped short.

'Look—a bride!' she exclaimed.

The bridal car awaited me. A new life awaited me. There was to be an elaborate wedding, a honeymoon in Spain and a move fifty miles from London to the Surrey town of Guildford.

I did not know, at that moment, that my simple ambitions of being a conventional wife and mother would not easily be achieved. That there would be times when my life would be far from conventional, and that my desire to produce a family would be frustrated by two miscarriages and the tragedy of a dead child.

I did not know then, that my emotions would range from the depths to the heights in the next few years and would eventually be expressed in the form of a book—written so that others might understand my experience.

As I stood framed in the doorway, on that September Sunday, traditionally clad in white satin, as so many brides before me, I was thankfully unaware of what lay ahead.

The middle-aged lady, eager and excited, rushed forward with her umbrella to escort me to the car.

'Mazel and brachas! (Good luck and blessings),' she cried. 'Mazel and brachas!'

My parents got into the car, and we sped away to the Synagogue.

The ceremony conducted in Hebrew, the partaking by my new husband, Michael, and myself of a sip of wine from a common goblet and the breaking of a glass underfoot were followed by a wedding party which was fairly typical of many Jewish weddings of that time. There was an emphasis on food and drink, mainly the former, exemplified by the menu of several courses, and punctuated by a sorbet in the middle to enable guests to eat the latter part of the meal with renewed appetite.

Traditional toasts were drunk to one and all, and lengthy orations, rightfully in praise of my parents, delivered.

Music and dancing were followed by tea and pastries.

It was an extravagant affair, which I would not have wished to change, although I cannot claim that the feeling was shared by Michael. In fact in subsequent years, he always referred to the occasion as 'your wedding'. Perhaps I should not have allowed my parents to waste their money on such an unproductive function. How much more sensible it would have been to invest it in the furnishing of our future home.

But every ship has the right to a bottle of champagne on its launching and I wanted to go out in style too.

'Look after the luxuries,' I told my friend, Ruth, who held the opposite view, 'and the necessities will look after themselves!'

Michael and I had met each other eighteen months before and although I would not go so far as to claim it was love at first sight, there was an immediate feeling of recognition of each other. I don't know what he saw in me, other than the carefully made up face and slim figure, for I had little else to offer a potential husband at that time. As he was fond of telling me in later years, an Eskimo simply wouldn't have taken on a wife with my lack of domestic skills and my abhorrence of sewing, and a secretarial training and several O-Levels simply would not have substituted. However I, in my first look at him, saw strength, kindness, and good humour in his eyes. I had in the past had a tendency to be attracted by rogues (haven't we all?), but here, for the first time, I thought I saw the father of my children. We gravitated to each other by common consent, and our engagement occurred a year later following a courtship that was not without its ups and downs. He was unpunctual and forgetful. I was self-centred and pretty spoiled, as well as being totally undomesticated. By the time we got married, he was nearly thirty and I was five years younger. We had already developed some sharp corners that required rubbing off.

As I walked down the aisle on my father's arm, I nearly stopped in my tracks and returned whence I came. Could this be the biggest mistake of my life? But the music played on and my feet carried on walking into marriage.

Delaying the commencement of reality still further, Michael and I flew off to Torremolinos, but like many young couples, we found the honeymoon an overrated experience and since we and most people in our hotel were soon incapacitated by a virulent Spanish germ, we were not left with many romantic memories of the holiday.

Married life began in earnest with our arrival at our house in Guildford—a two-bedroomed semi, with builder's yard attached, from where Michael ran a plumbing and heating business. This was ostensibly a temporary measure, since Michael had assured me that within about three months, we would be able to move into our dream house, in a delightful setting, tucked away on a country lane.

Shortly after we had become engaged, Michael had driven me into a village a few miles from the office/builders' yard, and in almost total darkness, had shown me a field where weeds and grass were practically waist high. He had been offered this secluded plot, with planning permission for a bungalow, by an architect-contact, and considered we were extremely lucky to have the opportunity to buy it.

There were modern estates springing up all over the country with new homes suitable for young marrieds. But Michael was not prepared to consider a home that came ready to use without any additional work required. Part of the charm of buying a new property was the prospect of knocking it about a bit. He had, for example, also expressed an interest in buying a mill, and had some fancy ideas about water running through the living room, contained in some sort of glass aqueduct. I was decidedly unenthusiastic about this and settled for the lesser of the two evils—a modern bungalow—in the back of beyond. So I gave the final assent, added most of my savings to his capital, and in no time, the legal wheels were grinding and the unkempt piece of land was ours.

Very few people realised how much I dreaded life in what seemed to me to be the heart of the country. I had after all lived for years in a main road in London, with the comforting noise of several buses stopping outside my front door, and all my working life had been spent in the West End, from Haymarket to Mayfair, where the nearest thing to countryside was Green Park.

Nevertheless, I tried to show enthusiasm for our potential home; many weekends during our engagement were spent at our wilderness, and a large mechanical digger was purchased in order to clear the land, the site of an old orchard.

The apple trees were all blighted, so we had to be ruthless. As a learner driver with two failed tests behind me, I might not have seemed the obvious choice of driver of the yellow monster, but I would probably have been even less use in dealing with the sprouting growth of all shapes and sizes. Each apple tree was attached by Michael to the digger, after which I, sitting high above him in my cab, operated the controls and yanked the tree, roots and all, from the earth like a stopper from a bottle. With much more effort, and reluctantly, an oak and a horse chestnut tree were removed too, and a mammoth bonfire was often the highlight of the day's efforts.

Fortunately, because I came to love the appearance of those huge mature trees, we were able to save three more oaks and two acacias, by moving the proposed position of the house.

Not one to miss an opportunity, Michael also employed the digger to excavate an enormous hole at the end of the garden, in order that we could one day build a swimming pool.

Michael had always wanted a house in the country with a circular drive, and I for my part, would be getting a modern house that should be relatively easy to run. But, when the wedding had taken place, the piece of land, looking somewhat smaller now it was devoid of its weeds and trees, was still quite naked of building.

It was therefore necessary for me to serve out my apprenticeship in housewifery at 'The Yard', as the men insisted on calling my first marital home, and indeed, few brides could have been more in need of training in that field than myself.

Michael, who was on the premises for a great part of the day, soon became aware of my inadequacies. I had always accused him of seeing me through 'rose-coloured spectacles', but if he had at any time imagined he was marrying the perfect woman, he was now sadly disillusioned.

I was a day-dreamer and found it difficult to get down to a type of work which was wholly unfamiliar to me. I had no routine. Sometimes I sat in the bath in the morning, becoming engrossed in cleaning the tiles or polishing the taps from that vantage point, while more noticeable areas of the house remained neglected.

I never knew which job to tackle first and whatever was eventually chosen as my priority would invariably leave some other area of chaos to be discovered.

Often I was summoned to make tea for several plumbers. Needless to say, one session of tea-making and washing up would set back my housework for hours, but since 'Women's Lib' had not yet made any impression on the world, I meekly accepted my humble role without protest.

I found cooking more stimulating than housework, though I had not yet acquired any great talent in the kitchen. However, my attempts at midday lunches were often frustrated by frequent interruptions from callers— salesmen, the team of plumbers, neighbours wanting to beg or borrow some small item from 'The Yard' or even borrow Michael himself to put in a light bulb, or gain access to an accidently locked house. Michael, unlike myself, could fit an incredible number of jobs into the working day, which rather accentuated my own lack of speed, at the same time confirming the fact that opposites really do attract.

Like many a new bride far from her parents, I was very homesick, and 'The Yard' in no way resembled a home. In addition, not only had I left behind in London most of my friends from both my school and working days, but also the Jewishness and warmth of my original neighbourhood. There was no-one here to wish me 'Mazel and brachas!'.

My immediate neighbours were elderly and vaguely disapproving of 'The Yard' on their very doorsteps, even while sometimes finding it useful to have a young man around. There was a constant stream of activity which Mrs Bird on one side would occasionally watch from a peephole in the fence; men in vans loading lavatory pans, and piles of pipes and fittings lying in heaps in the concrete garden. And where the 'front room' should have been was a dusty, untidy office which I did nothing to improve, and which housed Michael's young secretary, Maureen.

Maureen, a cheerful and friendly girl, had no hesitation in sabotaging my reputation amongst my curious neighbours, confirming that I never hung washing out in the back yard, and implying that I draped it over the radiators, (though I actually had an electric drying cabinet) and revealing to them other such horrendous domestic shortcomings, whilst disarmingly confessing to me that she did so.

In no way, could I become mistress of this abode. On the contrary, I was an intruder. The staff, and even the local people had become used to certain behaviour, which was not going to change simply because I had arrived on the scene. The local roadsweeper, I discovered after some time, used our outside loo, and Maureen and all the plumbers used my kitchen to make tea, (when I wasn't doing it) and wash their hands.

Recognising the advantages of removing myself from the scene, I went to a local agency and applied for a position as a temporary shorthand typist.

'Temps' in Guildford were apparently not so popular as the London variety, and it was a couple of months before I was given a job with Cow and Gate. My new job added nothing to my efficiency in the home. Flinging the bedclothes back to represent a passable imitation of a made bed, I would rush from the house and beg a lift into town from any of the plumbers available. After a few days, there was invariably a complaint from Michael that his toes were sticking out of the bottom of the bed.

Nevertheless, I settled into something of a routine at Cow

and Gate. I worked reasonably hard and was even offered a permanent job there. But far from typing letters to mothers about baby foods, it was my ambition to produce my own baby as soon as possible. At twenty-five I felt, rightly or wrongly that I had no time to lose. In any case, my mother had a history of miscarriages, and there was a vague fear at the back of my mind that I too might have problems.

As I began to find my feet at home, I made my first tentative attempts at entertaining. My mother-in-law, and my brother- and sisters-in-law, with their respective spouses and one fiancé were each invited to partake of Sunday lunch. The occasions were marked by general panic, Michael rushing around to assist in clearing-up operations and potato peeling and the like. One might have thought that my newly acquired brothers and sisters were a group of inspectors from the *Good Food Guide,* instead of a rather nice bunch of young people.

I was soon bold enough to ask my only local friend, Susan, and her husband to join us for an evening meal. Susan, a vivacious Irish blonde, had shared my office in London for a year, and had been a recognised 'kindred spirit' from the moment she had walked through the door. Now, fortuitously, she lived about six miles away with her husband Bruce, a quietly spoken surveyor from that same office, and their young baby.

This was the only occasion when I can recall actually feeling nauseous at my own cooking, although a crop of spots which appeared on the following day revealed that I had chicken-pox rather than food-poisoning.

Unfortunately, as a result of this, our regular trips to our parents had to be temporarily curtailed until the quarantine period was over. We still sought the warmth and welcome of our parents' homes, for we had not yet created a home for ourselves. We were still, after three or four months, two individuals full of obstinacy and dogmatic ideas, disappointed in each other's inadequacies. Michael's bouts of sarcasm frequently sparked off tears and tantrums in me. Living together for twenty-four hours a day only accentuated our differences, and I returned at last with relief to my letters on infant care and baby food.

Within a very few weeks, however, came the realisation that possibly I too, might be joining the ranks of worried mums writing for advice from the 'Medical Department' on the virtues of ground rice or chopped chicken. According to the calendar I must be pregnant.

It had all seemed so easy, it was difficult to believe it was true, but the pregnancy was duly confirmed and since the doctor was unconcerned about the chicken-pox attack in the early weeks, the next few months passed without problems.

In the middle of the pregnancy, we were able to spend a dreamy holiday in Djerba, off the coast of Tunisia, reputedly Ulysees' island of the lotus eaters.

This holiday was memorable only for the amount of time spent doing nothing, but in my pregnant state, it seemed ideal. Bedrooms at our hotel were lines of chalet bungalows served by a central dining room and various bars. In our case, we could step out on to an almost deserted beach, where few people could view my 'bulge' housed in a swimsuit. A small group of Bedouins were permanently stationed on the same beach, ready to hire out a horse or camel for a ride, but I at least did not feel obliged to do anything so energetic. The tensions of our honeymoon were gone and the pressures of fractious infants were yet to come.

By night we sat and occasionally danced in the hotel club. Often I felt the early movements of my child, strangely awakened by the beat of the music.

But just as Ulysses' men were dragged reluctantly from their idle pleasures, we too soon had to face reality once again. Reality that included my new temporary job in an accountant's office, a lack of money in the bank, an unbuilt bungalow and a house that was very far from being a home.

Unto Us

Possibly one of the least practical things that Michael ever did was to marry me in 1966, not two years after he had invested most of his money in a new business. Two may live as cheaply as one, for all I know, but not when they venture into the purchase of land. For all the money we had saved and some we didn't even have, had been spent on that bare expanse of land, and now as the months rolled by, our efforts were devoted to filling up the increasingly huge chasm that was our overdraft. My somewhat mean salary went straight into that seemingly bottomless pit, never to be seen again. Any additional money spent on building was a drain on our meagre resources, so at first it was limited to making use of the talents of our plumbing team during slack times. In the winter of 1966, they laid a solid new layer of road on to the muddy footpath leading to 'the site' as we called it, so that in the course of the next few months, heavy lorries could deliver their loads of pipes, bricks, cement and so on.

Our present home was sparsely furnished and lacking in frills for we begrudged every penny spent on our premises at the office. We abided by a policy of 'make do and mend' and had acquired from our families a couple of old armchairs, a gate-leg table and some unwanted strips of stair carpet to furnish our living quarters.

I always welcomed our trips to London, the cosiness of my parents' home, and the return to my roots. Sometimes it was possible to see my old school-friend Ruth, who also made such periodic excursions to visit her mother and freckle-faced student sister, Rita.

Ruth, a slim dignified girl with auburn glints in her hair, who had married a month before me, was now, like me, expecting her first baby in the autumn. Our friendship of fifteen years' standing was impeded by the distance between us, for she had moved some fifty miles away from home to Maidstone, and our occasional visits to each other involved a long drive. Nevertheless, we and another school-friend, Pam, persuaded our husbands to take us on these trips when we could, inspecting with interest each other's first domestic efforts. Ruth and Pam had each acquired newly built estate houses, which I viewed with a pang of envy, despite all sophisticated comment about 'little boxes'. Our bungalow, when completed, would no doubt be just as neat and immaculate, but that event seemed far in the future, and in any case, I had no idea how I would adjust to country life and was happy to put it out of my mind.

In the last couple of months of my pregnancy, our journeyings ceased. I gave up my job to make preparation for the great day. Despite my lack of enthusiasm for housework, it was my intention to spring-clean, for the house would no doubt be neglected during the early months of the baby's life. I had no romantic illusions about motherhood. I would feel a flutter of fear at the thought of the baby's birth, in spite of the course of relaxation classes I had attended, and as to its eventual presence in my life, I could really only imagine it yelling, particularly in the middle of the night. So in a way, I set rather a great value on those last two months. They were the end of an era, as had been the end of my single life, and in addition, I felt they were the end of my freedom, for perhaps the next fifteen or twenty years.

Consequently, I felt rather cheated when Michael's secretary, Maureen, broke her arm within three days of the end of my employment. For a full month, my secretarial skills were needed in the office, and then there was only one month left and so many things to do and to buy.

I had a list, which weighed heavily on my conscience, issued by the hospital, with orders to bring nighties, bath towel, a crepe bandage, a piece of old linen and other faintly eccentric items. But by the time I eventually made the trip into Guildford for my purchases, there was a mere week left before the Expected Day of Arrival.

In spite of waking with a backache, I could not postpone the pilgrimage any longer and Michael left me in the town centre before he himself set out for London. Having been remarkably fit during the whole of the pregnancy, I was irritated now at the thought that I might be plagued with backache for a whole week until the baby was born. But as the day progressed and my acquisitions grew heavier, the backache too increased in severity. In my innocence, I had not imagined that the baby would be born early, but I now realised that my labour was imminent. Even so, I frenziedly continued my search—nappy bucket—pins— roller towel material—(what could they possibly want with that?) and eventually I caught a bus home right in the middle of the rush hour, not even having the good sense to get a taxi. Determined to get a seat, on this day of all days, I placed myself and stomach squarely in front of a seated male and my pointed look (and rounded tum) had the desired effect.

On my arrival home, I hurriedly packed my suitcase. Then, lonely and desolate in the empty house, aware of the first regular contractions, I sat wondering what to do next. I was afraid too, afraid of unknown pain, afraid of the adventure I must face entirely on my own.

In the next three hours, my sense of isolation remained unabated and indeed aggravated by the maternity home's reluctance to receive me. There was no sign of Michael, who had anticipated a late arrival home from London, and the only neighbour who had befriended me had herself been taken into hospital a few days before. Even my mother who telephoned during the course of the evening, could not become my confidante on this occasion. If I had told her I was in labour and on my own, she would have worried all night.

On a sudden inspiration I telephoned Susan, whom I recalled I had invited to tea on the following day, and she promptly drove over to escort me to the maternity home.

Before leaving home, I rang my mother-in-law to see if Michael had called in on his way home. I had the satisfaction of delivering my dramatic news to my mother-in-law with a calmness I did not feel. Michael was immediately dispatched homewards, to share some part of the night with me.

And a long and lonely night it was, slightly mitigated by

Michael's stay at my side for two or three hours, and a restless slumber induced by an injection in the early hours of the morning. Michael was dismissed at this point and with obvious relief returned home to get some sleep himself. He was completely out of his element in a situation where there was nothing he could physically do to improve it.

I awoke some time before dawn, writhing and tossing just like a character in a television drama. It was the worst moment of labour, for once in the delivery room, the contractions were hardly strong enough to encourage me to push.

'You're wasting the contractions,' bemoaned the nurse, and suddenly I remembered that babies must not take too long actually being born. I glanced at the clock and saw that I had been in the delivery room for nearly an hour.

Soon they'll get out the forceps, I thought. And I pushed!

'That's it! That's it! Come on!' exhorted the nurse.

And suddenly with a slithering sensation, my baby was born and I saw his tiny silhouette, as the nurse held him aloft; and then he was in my arms, a small round bundle with a screwed up face.

My son Robert.

Muddling Along

Motherhood did not come to me with a great burst of maternal emotions. Sad to say, my initial feelings were far more related to pride in having done the production job without too much fuss, than any great love for the small human being who purported to be a very close relation.

I was surprised at the frequency with which he was presented to me for feeding and I did not immediately warm to this time-consuming stranger, for I had difficulty believing in my role as mother to him.

Nevertheless, as I got to know him, I was full of admiration for him, for he blossomed before my eyes, and showed signs of becoming a beautiful baby. I had never been a lover of babies as a group. Nor had I really known any as individuals, and my expectations were low. It came as something of a surprise to me therefore to find that I had produced what must surely be the most perfect baby in the world. During the day, he lay in a cot at the foot of my bed. Most of the time he slept contentedly, and there was rarely a tear from him.

I took full advantage of the fairly leisurely time in the maternity home, which remained so until the seventh day of my stay, when I received instruction in the skills of nappy changing and baby bathing, with a carte blanche to try them out on my own squirming infant. I was also told to make my own bed with the help of the nurse, and this was a rather rude awakening. By the time I was finished, I was puffing and blowing after the strenuous effort. But it had one great advantage: I learned how to make 'hospital corners' and I became quite obsessional about them after that. Michael's toes never poked out of the bottom of the bed again.

I had arranged to stay with my parents on my departure from the maternity home. However, when I mentioned this fact,

I fell foul of Sister, who it seemed had already summed me up as idle and immature.

'You can't go gallivanting off to London with a young baby,' she told me.

She must have had some vision of me doing the rounds of nightclubs, theatres and parties, and I didn't know how to convince her that I really wasn't going to gallivant, just to be cared for by my own mother while I mastered the complicated skills of mothercraft.

I enjoyed my return to my own territory with baby Robert, who maintained his placid behaviour pattern. True, he awoke in the night for his feeds, which I considered to be a form of Chinese torture, but this could not be classed as naughtiness. My two married sisters-in-law, Sonia and Karla, each with a son of their own, assured me I was extremely lucky to have such a contented baby.

Nevertheless, once we arrived back in Guildford, I suffered from total exhaustion, causing me to fall asleep after the six a.m. feed and awake to discover the office below my bedroom full of activity and noise and Robert all ready for the ten o'clock feed.

Day after day, I muddled through the baths, feeds and nappy changes, finding little time for anything else, for the carrying out of these tasks seemed enormously time-consuming. Any faint resemblance to a routine was based on a suggestion from my old school friend Pam: 'Look after the baby, feed the family, keep up with the washing and don't worry about anything else.'

It was difficult to obey the last order, but I knew her set of priorities were correct, and Robert, sleepy and well satisfied after each feed, was the proof of the pudding.

Only one cloud marred his otherwise untroubled babyhood, when at six weeks old, he developed an ugly breast abscess. After a week of antibiotics, this was removed by general anaesthetic, and special tiny equipment had to be brought into the casualty department where the operation took place. The nurses made a great fuss of baby Robert when he was brought in during the next few days; they said they were used to seeing much bigger children with scrapes on their knees.

Despite the varying times of my arrival at the casualty department for dressings of the wound, the receptionist was brisk but sympathetic. Her conversation suggested she imagined the baby was playing me up, and I perpetuated that injustice, rather than admit that I just couldn't get up in the mornings, after the dreadful night feeds.

The whole abscess episode was a bit of a nuisance, disrupting what little routine I had. But I didn't really worry about Robert, because I'd heard so many times what hardy creatures babies are. Four years later, I had cause to doubt that generalisation, and remembered wryly my simple faith that all would be well.

The months went by and we progressed through breast feeding to mixed feeding and from incisors to molars and still Robert was happy. Now he chose to eat at more civilised times and we all breakfasted together on boiled eggs. The days of the hurried slice of toast in a vertical position were over. We had become a family!

Despite a large and well justified inferiority complex about my inability to run the home, I felt I had made a fairly successful job of bringing up the baby, and for the first time in my married life, I gained some confidence. Baby Robert appeared to be a credit to me, and Michael often said, 'I always knew you'd be a good mother'.

But although I spent much time reading articles on babies, on aspects of feeding and weaning, teething and toilet training, I did not really build a relationship with Robert when he was a tiny baby. Perhaps I would have been better advised to put away the books and get down on the floor to play with him, but I was too guilty about my inadequacies as a housewife to spend time in the enjoyment of play.

It was Michael who had a special relationship with Robert. As the oldest of four children, Michael was totally at ease in the presence of little ones. Immediately recognised by small boys as a 'romper' and 'rough-and-tumbler', and by larger boys as the sort of uncle-figure who would allow them to help with pasting, tarring or whitewashing jobs, he could in addition communicate with this foot-long creature, at present devoid of any appreciable powers of mobility or conversation. He would pick the little boy up with two hands and, holding him a few inches away from his face, would address him solemnly, carefully articulating his words.

'Say, "Dad-dy, Dad-dy".'

And the baby, no more than a few months old, would watch goggle-eyed and form shapes with his mouth in imitation or response.

In time, he learned to recognise the pale blue Wolseley which Michael drove and would shriek with delight at the sight of his father approaching, and howl at his often speedy departure, en route to another job.

When Robert was in the middle of his first year, the plumbing business began to take up more of my time. Michael's secretary had left and one of the plumbers had been installed in the front office. In theory, he would be a clerk-cum-emergency plumber. In practice, there were so many emergencies that the telephone rang incessantly calling him away, while the bookkeeping ground to a halt.

For the next few months, I answered the telephone a couple of dozen times a day, and became an expert on ball valves and leaks, often advising panicking housewives to turn the water off at the stopcock, and make a small hole in the ceiling, to prevent the ceiling coming down. I don't suppose a single housewife ever took notice of my advice and while I dispensed it, Robert sat poised—mid-bosom (mine) or bare-bottomed (his) awaiting my attention.

Luckily for me during this period, Robert had an easy going temperament. He had become an attractive baby with dark curls, blue-green eyes and a dimple in one cheek. It was a period in his life I later looked back on with nostalgia, for his personality had developed, but he was not yet old enough or accomplished enough to be mischievous. He would speed from room to room on all fours but his agility had not yet become a source of danger. Sometimes he rode on Michael's shoulders, sitting proudly, his back erect like a young horseman, surveying the scene around him. But he was happy to sit in the pram too, watching traffic and people passing by. Indeed because of his shrieks of joy when he recognised a familiar face, he made more friends than I had amongst the local people. Both my elderly neighbours were to be seen talking to him from time to time and in fact, he created a small feeling of warmth between them and me, which had not previously existed.

Our neighbours on one side had never had any children, whilst the elderly couple, the Birds, on the other side, had a handicapped son of around forty. Like Robert, he was always outside watching the world on fine days, and was tanned and as fit as he could be in the circumstances. Once, the Queen went through our street on her way to the Queen Elizabeth Barracks not far away and gave Gerald a special wave.

We were sad to hear one day that he had died. Michael and one of the plumbers, Reg, who lived two doors away, went to the funeral, and I, with trepidation in my heart, felt it was incumbent upon me to visit the mourners very soon afterwards. They had devoted their lives to him and the reason for my reluctance was because I imagined I would have to face some sort of emotional scene. Perhaps I recognised even then the poignancy of the death of a child during the lifetime of its parents.

Despite my lack of rapport with my neighbours and my fears of embarrassment, I could not let the occasion pass without acknowledging Gerald's death. This would set up a barrier between us and my embarrassment at any later meeting would have been all the greater.

I knocked on the kitchen door (it was not usual for neighbours to use the front doors) and was welcomed in. I was surprised at how glad they were to see me. They gave me a sherry and showed me letters and talked about Gerald. They were relaxed, and even happy, perhaps, because he had not outlived them, and would never have to spend his days in a place where he was not loved. Far from being hysterical, they were very glad to talk about him. I recognised with satisfaction that I had made the right decision.

By this time, we had lived in our so-called temporary home for well over a year. I wasted little time now on worrying about how I would adjust to living in the country, for I really wondered whether the dream bungalow would ever be completed.

The laying of foundations had appeared to be a slow process, for much work was carried out under the ground. Twelve courses of bricks were laid and drain pipes put in place, followed by hardcore and a waterproof layer, but at the end of the first year's work, all that could be seen was a rectangular slab covered in concrete.

Then came a much more exciting era when the bricklayer, Mr Dean arrived and laid brick on brick with speed and skill, and within a few weeks there were walls and window frames, and we could walk giggling through the various holes which would become door ways, and point to the kitchen and bedrooms.

All our visiting friends and relations were taken on a tour of the site until it became quite a bore, and still, as far as I was concerned, totally divorced from reality. The reality was our bare little semi, with its dusty corners, secondhand armchairs and uncarpeted bedrooms. The luxuries we would enjoy in our future home were a pipe dream—in which I did not really believe.

Whenever we had visitors, its drabness was accentuated, and despite the usual frenzied burst of tidying and polishing, at the end of the activity, I could always see it clearly for what it was.

However, we were not unhappy there. We had made it a home, albeit an unglamorous one, and it was only when I looked at it with the critical eyes of an outsider that I found real dissatisfaction with it.

While Robert was a baby, we were still fairly mobile. Visiting our friends, our parents in London and the in-laws was a major part of our social life.

When money became tight, we ceased to run the Wolseley

and drove to our visits in one of the vans, installing pram, high chair, and other baby paraphernalia in its convenient empty back.

Once we returned from a trip to Ruth and Roger, after Michael's company had installed heating in their home, in an undignified 'pick-up' lorry, in order to bring back spare copper pipe, only to run out of petrol a hundred yards from home. We made a pretty picture, no doubt, marching up the hill with copper pipe on our shoulders, and carry cot being ferried along too, Michael striding along at the front and I scurrying along behind, with expressions respectively of amusement and irritation.

There was often an element of ridiculousness in our travels, like the time when we hired a car to attend a function and found ourselves resplendent in dinner jacket and long evening dress faced with a puncture with no jack. Michael dealt with the situation by borrowing some marble stone from a funeral director opposite and driving the car up on to it, to change the wheel.

I used to rely upon Michael's ingenuity, just as he came eventually to rely upon my attention to detail. Other people too would call on him. Ruth's sister, Rita rang for help when we were in London one weekend, saying she was stranded at Euston Station with all the acquisitions and leftovers from a term at University, and since I had always regarded her with a mixture of the somewhat patronising superiority and affection of an older sister, we went to her rescue and delivered her and her accumulated possessions to her home.

Early in 1968, Michael's youngest sister, Philippa, followed her brothers and sister into matrimony. We left Robert with my two closest aunts for the occasion, since my parents were with us at the wedding. The Aunties were delighted to look after the baby whom they adored, but their pleasure was tinged with sadness, for in an adjoining room, my uncle lay seriously ill.

A few weeks later my uncle died, leaving unfulfilled his dream of spending his retirement at his favourite resort.

My aunts sadly packed up and moved into the already purchased house in Hove, near Brighton. Not long after, my parents, lonely without their close family, followed suit. My last link with the home of my childhood was severed.

Housey-Housey

Three winters had passed since we first stood by the swaying grasses at the site of our future home, and we were still 'living above the shop'. The bungalow was still incomplete, but considerable progress had been made. The roof was on, the garage was complete with doors, but a large amount of work still remained on the inside. The plastering, glazing and what is known as 'second fixing' (when pipes are linked to basins, wires connected to switches and cupboards inserted) still had to be carried out.

Except for the plumbing and central heating, all the other tradesmen, with such quaint names as the Sparks, the Chippie and the Spread, were called in from the outside, and the length of time between each trade depended upon the amount of money presently in the kitty, for needless to say, we were constantly short of money; the business was subsidising the bungalow. The bridging loan (for use in building the house) was supporting the business. The Bank Manager was frequently lecturing, but Peter often had to be robbed to pay Paul.

Our business had expanded rapidly, but we did not have sufficient capital to finance the large contracts we had taken on. Payment from our main contractors was so slow that we could not afford the large weekly wage bills. On many weeks the tension mounted as we wondered if the wage cheque would be cleared. Once I drew the last ten or twenty pounds from my post office account, which many women secretly keep, to help pay the wages.

In addition to our financial problems, a new delaying factor in our home-building was rearing an extremely ugly head. There was no mains electricity available at the site of the bungalow and cable would need to be laid along the rough foot path access to the site. The local military gentleman who owned this footpath, and who had shown no distress or even interest at our improving its condition, now put in a claim for compensation for its disturbance. But although it would have been reinstated to its present condition, the compensation offered by the Electricity Board was refused by him, and he stated that it was not just a matter of money. It was a matter of principle!

We were certainly not prepared to offer him money ourselves in order to discover the depth of his principles. The problem was academic at the moment, but at the backs of our minds was a feeling that we should be prepared for battle.

But as, in spite of the lack of electricity, it really did look as if the end was in sight, we decided to put our semi, with builder's yard attached, on the market.

A few potential buyers drifted in to view the far from palatial home, in the hope of setting up a new business, for the permission to carry out certain trades or businesses was one of the property's main assets. But because of the residential surroundings, we had to reject offers from people involved in a number of noisy trades and we ended up with one apparently genuinely interested visitor who wanted to turn the place into a market garden, but who had difficulty obtaining the money she needed.

With the immediate prognosis on all fronts rather unsatisfactory, we contemplated the least logical step of all—another baby.

I had not in the fifteen month period since Robert was born, developed any greater affection for the race of new babies. In fact I found that bringing up a toddler was in itself quite a time-consuming occupation. As soon as Robert had learned to stand and had made his first tentative efforts to walk around holding on to the furniture, he had become a hazard. As he progressed round the room, small tables would be in danger of being over-thrown and hanging tablecloths, stacked with crockery, yanked to the floor.

Our staircase was steep and I had taught him to crawl down on his front but if ever I saw him poised at the top of the stairs, I was afraid he would topple down the entire flight, though he never did. It was an age at which I could not let him out of my sight and most of the time, he accompanied me round the house as I worked. He rarely played with toys, being a sociable child who preferred the company of people. I used to talk to him non-stop, but sometimes I longed for a reprieve and would imprison him in his playpen for a short respite. I imagined that a new baby would soon become a companion for him, so for me, the decision to become pregnant now was a cold-blooded one based on my opinion that Robert's brother or sister should be two years his junior. The financial and other considerations we assumed and hoped were merely transient problems, and in any case, Robert had made very little difference to our financial situation. Baby baths and carry-cots were freely passed around the family and little boys' clothes frequently handed down the line.

In addition, Robert was an adaptable child, quite accustomed to the office activity, and fitting easily into our disorganised life style. Was it possible that our second child would follow the same pattern?

Initially, indeed it did. Just like Robert, it was conceived with startling immediacy, and calculations revealed that its birth would occur in October, the very month of Robert's second birthday. We were impressed at our own cleverness and happily told the family the glad tidings.

For some time, Michael had tried to awaken some spark of enthusiasm in me for the slowly growing bungalow. He suggested I leaf through glossy magazines, but I told him I had my own ideas about the decor and didn't need to look at magazines. This was partly true, but my refusal was also a great deal to do with my feeling of disbelief that we would ever really move into the bungalow, and my fearful and unspoken desire to maintain the status quo, in spite of its shortcomings. For this reason, I had made no real effort to obtain a driving licence, other than suffering a few trial lessons with Michael. These had proved conclusively to me that I would never learn to drive with him at my elbow, issuing commands and rhetorical questions:

'Why are you driving at forty miles per hour in second gear?' 'Why are you driving at twenty miles per hour in fourth gear?' (I considered that being in the correct gear was additional to, rather than part of, good driving.) 'Why aren't you driving five feet from the kerb?'

Michael was concerned at my lack of interest in this facet of country living, warning me time and time again that I would feel very cut off in the country if I couldn't drive.

When he arrived home one day, asking me to choose paint colours for the various room, I knew it was no longer possible to regard the move as some nebulous future happening. At last I knew in my heart that the time was drawing close.

Apart from Michael's fruitless efforts, I had also had the dubious benefit of inadequate driving instruction when I was eighteen years old (and had consequently failed my driving test twice). Now, I felt it was necessary to acquire an instructor of experience and good repute and of calm and authoritative manner. Joan, the wife of one of our plumbers, Reg, who lived two doors away, had recently passed her driving test. She had been taught by a retired police instructor, a Mr Oliver. He seemed to fill the bill entirely and had, in addition, as do most professional instructors, the advantage of not being emotionally involved with me. Slowly, some of the rules of the road began to penetrate.

Soon, we had filled the bungalow with pastels of various shades, green, blue, pink and lilac, with the pleasant knowledge that these simple decisions were far from irrevocable. Now, with the bungalow nearly habitable, it was time to enquire whether we could receive our mortgage. We had held a bridging loan since the commencement of building. Together with our business overdraft, the money we owed had grown to some phenomenal sum. We knew the Bank Manager would be quite relieved to see some part of it paid back. There was the problem of the electricity, or lack of it, however.

Michael decided to make some general enquiries.

'Would a person be granted a mortgage,' he asked on the telephone, 'if he generated his own electricity?'

(He had actually acquired a paraffin-run generator from a scrap yard, which didn't as yet work, but there was always the possibility that it might, given time.

'Oh, no, sir,' came the reply. 'We couldn't possibly grant a mortgage without mains electricity.'

Here was cause for real concern. With resignation we learned from the building society, in due course that they would send their representative to inspect the completed property, when he would undoubtedly learn the worst. We suggested that he first telephoned us in order that we might direct him there. Soon, we heard that their representative had attempted to inspect the property, but had been unable to find it. Patiently, we advised them once again—we were happy to direct their man to the site, which was very difficult to find, hidden as it was in the woods, if he would care to ring us when he was intending to attempt to inspect again.

We never did hear from him—only a sheaf of papers arrived telling us our mortgage had been granted. We were quite hysterical with delight and amusement—and amazement! The Bank Manager must have been thrilled too.

We never did find out if anyone had actually inspected the bungalow. Was it carelessness, laziness, or maybe someone turning a blind eye? At any rate it had made a lot of difference to us that day.

Disappointments

I was hurrying frantically around a large department store, full of people. Or perhaps it was more like an oriental bazaar. I was desperately searching for a doctor— I was losing my baby! I knew I had to lie down and put my feet up. But there was no place to lie down and no-one to help me.

Relief flooded over me when I realised I was in bed dreaming, until in my fully wakened state, the nagging ache at the pit of my stomach told me that the dream was coming true.

I panicked; I wept hysterically when I told Michael and he could only react with impatience; he sent me back to bed and soon Robert joined me in the room. But I didn't really want him there—I was too worried about myself; I couldn't call upon my normal reserves of patience, necessary for dealing with little boys of eighteen months.

Later in the day, I crept downstairs and telephoned Joan, as well as trying the doctor for a second time. Joan came over and promised to give Robert lunch, and later Michael came in and found her armed with the carpet sweeper, tidying up the living room, in case the doctor came, for I was still an awful housewife. He was unbelievably angry; he was a very independent person. I found it very annoying that, when he was not in a position to give me constant help, he couldn't understand my seeking help elsewhere. He didn't seem to understand that women with small children do help each other. But independent people seem to be so unbending in this respect. It did rather add to my misery to have to argue with him on this point. He also didn't really seem to regard my possible miscarriage as of major importance.

The doctor too, appeared to be fairly unperturbed; a couple of days' rest and possibly all would be well, he told me.

So I stayed miserably abed until things returned to normal, then warily returned to my disorganised existence. But soon relief made me almost complacent and I was full of plans for the next few weeks. After Robert's birth, I had imagined myself to be a fairly healthy young woman who would not have problems such as my mother had experienced. In spite of my doctor's statement that two out of five women spontaneously miscarry in the early part of pregnancy, it was a blow to my pride to find that I might after all be vulnerable in this respect. It was restricting not to be able to behave normally and I did not really want to believe in the necessity for restraint. On one or two occasions, I rebelliously flouted the authoritative voice of common sense that told me what to do and what not to do. Just once, I carried my heavy standard typewriter into a warm room to do some typing, assuring myself that such a small thing could do no damage.

In the middle of April, a couple of weeks after the first warning, I haemorrhaged. Fearful and depressed, I waited for a doctor, who arrived after two or three hours and sent for an ambulance immediately.

The ambulance men had quite a job carrying me down our steep steps, but they tried to cheer me up, making jokes as we went along. When I was finally in the ambulance, Michael told Robert to go and kiss Mummy 'Bye-Bye.' He was a pathetic sight. He'd been suffering from an infection that he couldn't shake off and he looked thin and dirty and neglected. He said 'Bye-Bye, Mummy,' but I could tell he didn't really understand what was going on. It was the first time I'd ever left him for more than a couple of hours and, as the ambulance drove off, I shed a few tears at the thought of his bewilderment at this incomprehensible situation.

The ambulance men left me at the hospital gate, while they got permission for me to enter. No doubt such formalities are necessary even in the direst of emergencies! However, with permission granted, I was wheeled into a ward where a nun was preparing a bed for me.

'I've warmed it up for you,' she told me. It was deliciously cosy and comforting. I remembered then how after Robert was born a nun came and gently washed me and then sat by me for at least a quarter of an hour mopping my brow whilst I was stitched. Such small kindnesses are not forgotten.

The doctor, a pleasant, good looking young man, arrived soon. I appreciated his directness when he told me that I would have a 'D and C' very shortly. I had had little hope that the baby would be saved, and I felt a certain amount of relief that I was receiving hospital care and not allowed to miscarry at home, as one of my neighbours had only recently.

Anaesthetics had improved greatly since I had last had a minor operation ten years before. I still remembered the mask that smelled of rubber being placed on my face and the nausea afterwards. I was relieved to find now that a small injection made me quite relaxed and hazy. I was wheeled off somewhere where a lot of people were standing around in green overalls with masks over their mouths.

'Have you any children?' said one of the figures.

'Yes, a little boy of eighteen months.'

They asked me to count and I started, but I couldn't finish.

A hospital is a strange little world on its own, where perspectives are changed quite drastically. I spent only a few days there, but my feelings were distorted by the conditions of that particular world. On the one hand, by virtue of that unwritten law that says your husband shall visit you at seven thirty p.m., I felt desperately deprived, for Michael was conspicuous by his absence.

On the other hand, in a ward where women had parted with large sections of their female organs and walked around appearing to hold together what was left of their stomachs, I could not but regard my three-month miscarriage as rather trivial.

I awoke on the first day after the 'scrape' to realise with dismay that I had left at home, amongst other things, my contact lenses, my glasses, pants, dressing gown and purse. Without these things I was quite desperate. The person in the opposite bed was a blur and it is impossible to talk to a blur. I was wearing a hospital gynaecological ward nightie, which flapped open at the back like an apron, revealing a bare behind, so that I couldn't walk around the ward without a dressing gown; and without money, I could make no contact with the outside world. I was completely imprisoned. In vain did I try to telephone Michael reversing the charges. He was not there, and the automatic answering machine could not make the decision to accept my call.

Finally, I reached Joan, by reversing the charges to her home and entreated her to get Michael to deliver these essentials to me without delay. But in the end, it was kindhearted Joan, herself, who brought them, for Michael once again had had to rush off somewhere. He didn't visit me at all whilst I was in hospital and my feeling of humiliation was enormous.

Thinking back, I suppose it didn't seem awfully important to Michael, for I was only in hospital for two or three days, but to me it seemed I had been abandoned. Without money and with only female visitors, I wondered how many of my fellow occupants thought I was a potential unmarried mother who had deliberately caused her own abortion. At any rate, I saw myself as I assumed they saw me; as a woman whose man did not love her.

Logic told me that Michael was particularly busy. He had to make a hundred mile trip to Colchester which had already been planned. A drive to Brighton to deliver Robert into the care of my parents had been an added burden. But other thoughts refused to be driven from my head—he had rejected me because I had failed him. I had failed as a woman. I had failed to carry his child. I couldn't manage to get on with the simple job of producing a baby without causing general inconvenience all round. To this day, I could not say how much those thoughts were irrational nonsense; wasn't there a grain of truth contained in them?

But Michael was not an analytical person. He was not aware of such thoughts revolving round my own head and doubted the need for my reassurance during such a short period of time.

On the last day of my stay, I was partially mollified by the arrival of a bouquet of flowers from Michael, but as this was rather out of character, I assumed he had been given a little push in the right direction by Joan.

When the time came to depart, I hoped to show off my muscular husband, just to prove he really existed, but even then I was thwarted. He had to go away for the day and he asked Joan and Reg to pick me up.

The Sister in charge briskly sent me packing.

'Look after yourself, dear. Finish off your iron tablets and come to Outpatients in six weeks' time.'

Once released from hospital, the problems changed like a kaleidoscope.

First, we had to collect Robert from Brighton and initially, I was rejected by him, for he could not understand why I had deserted him. It was two hours before he would come to me.

I longed to stay with my parents and be coddled again as when I was a child, but Michael said, 'I need you at home. You've been away long enough.'

Only now in my own home, away from the brave bunch of women recovering from major surgery did my worries about Michael become scaled down to size, whilst at the same time, I recognised the extent of my own loss. I was angry and disappointed at the waste of time and waste of love and care that, in my way, I had given to the being within me from the moment I was aware of its presence, and I couldn't wait to become pregnant again. My second pregnancy had been the consequence of planning. My third pregnancy would be the result of deep longing.

We had returned to the mixture as before, but our house was now even less congenial than it had been. During the past few months, Michael had acted impulsively on a suggestion by our market garden lady and carried out a small conversion of our kitchen. Only when the work had been completed, halving the size of my kitchen, did we discover dismally that it was unlikely that our prospective purchaser would ever get access to the money she needed to buy our house.

So the house remained unsold. At the bungalow our electrical wrangles continued; and we didn't even have a new baby to look forward to. We both needed a break from this pattern of general inability to advance. It seemed a good moment to scrape up all available money and take a holiday.

At the end of May, I revisited the hospital. By that time, the urgent desire to be pregnant again had abated a little, despite the recent birth of a son to my sister-in-law, Philippa. Nevertheless, I was disappointed to be told to wait a while before trying again for a baby.

We tried to put our problems behind us and a few days later, we departed for our holiday. Romania had been recommended to us by our travel agent as being an economical place to go, in view of our usual impecuniousness. The weather could be expected to be good at this time of year.

In the event, it was just like an English seaside resort in the height of summer. Some days it poured, some days it drizzled and other days a thin sunshine broke through the overcast sky and we sat watching Robert make mud pies on the damp and chilly beach.

It was not an enjoyable holiday, though we made the best of it. There was a closed-in atmosphere that I didn't like; whispered hints of secret police and bugging of telephones; grim-faced officials in dark glasses occasionally to be seen speeding down the length of the beach in black Mercedes cars, and propaganda mixed with music, broadcast to the beach through loudspeakers.

There was a lack of freedom of choice which we found noticeably different from other holidays—an insistence on the guests sitting four to a table at the restaurant, rather like a regimented school party, and the presentation for two or three days of the same meat, so that we assumed we must eat the whole animal, before starting on a different one. There were ridiculous irritations, like having to sign a form confessing we had broken an ashtray in our room.

We were unregretful when the time came to leave the country, though we were twice held up at passport checkpoints because of trivial misunderstandings. At one point, left without a boarding card through no fault of my own, I really thought I would be stranded in this claustrophobic country, while the plane took off for England.

However, England welcomed us to her shores eventually with traditional fog, and since we were diverted unexpectedly to Gatwick Airport, we sought refuge with my parents in Brighton to recover from the ill-fated holiday.

Out of the Frying Pan?

Nothing had changed. Nothing had changed fundamentally after the miscarriage; and *still* nothing had changed, and suddenly it was impossible to live like that any longer.

I can't remember who said it first; I only know that in the course of one evening, we came to a sudden conclusion. We couldn't wait any longer for other people to make decisions that affected our lives. We would move into our bungalow—with or without electricity!

The next three weeks would be fairly busy. An inspection of the bungalow reminded us that there were many things to buy and do.

Dogmatically, I stated, 'I am *not* bringing an eighteen month old child to live on bare concrete floors.' There had been no point in fitting wood flooring to the concrete screed, as we had always intended to have fitted carpets. So carpets were a priority on our list of purchases. Furniture and furnishings, too, were required. There was no possibility of adapting our present curtains (machined by my own fair hand) to the large picture windows in the bungalow, thank goodness; and the thought of transferring our secondhand armchairs to this brand new home was too awful to consider.

Surprisingly, there was a lot of cleaning to do; dust lay everywhere in the new house—concrete dust which built up day by day and had to be damped down frequently, and sawdust caused by the carpentry work in the bedrooms and kitchen.

It was agreed that I would spend two weeks at my parents' house in Hove, during which time I would shop in Brighton and commute to the bungalow periodically to clean and prepare it. Robert would then be able to enjoy the benefits of the seaside, without my company. I was careful to explain this to him, however, as I did not want him to feel rejected as he had during my miscarriage.

First, however, I had to take my driving test, so much more important now—in view of the impending move.

I had more confidence now; no worries any longer about the mechanics of gear changing—and there was certainly no chance of my going through a red light, as I had done on my first, or was it my second test, when I was eighteen. Nevertheless, I was horribly nervous, as certain people always are when faced with an examiner in the flesh. If only I could have done a written paper on the subject.

My examiner was a tall pleasant looking man, the chief examiner, so Mr Oliver told me afterwards.

'He's always scrupulously fair,' he said, when I sadly told him the result of my test.

'You're not quite up to test standard,' the examiner had stated. I had not disgraced myself and Mr Oliver was not displeased with me, but I was bitterly disappointed. I had so hoped to pass, and now I would be marooned in the country, totally reliant on the hourly bus service—or my feet—at least until I could take the test again.

For a fortnight, however, I became a busy commuter, travelling to and fro—from our old home and new home to London and Brighton. I explored all the shops. In a Brighton store with Robert squalling with boredom in the background, I chose a beautiful green brocade curtain material which would blend with the pale green walls in the lounge. At the bungalow, I swept the rooms over and over again and patiently lined cupboards and drawers with brightly coloured paper. At the end of a day in London, I found myself marooned at Victoria Station by a train strike and was inspired to ring my mother-in-law for a night's lodging; only to find that Michael too was in London that night and together we drove home in the van.

Together in Guildford for the first time for days, we took the opportunity on the following day, to go to choose a traditional three-piece suite.

Then back I went once again to Hove to reassure my son that I had not after all deserted him again.

Naturally, the weather was at its tempting best, but, with all these other necessary activities summoning me, I only dared spend one or two afternoons at the seafront with Robert and my family.

One call in particular had to be made in Brighton, and that was to the head offices of the Electricity Board. Perhaps meeting me face to face, they would be persuaded to expedite the provision of our electricity supplies. As an added incentive, I took Robert in his pushchair, but got so tangled up with their revolving doors on my first abortive trip there, that I opted for a less pathetic approach on my second visit.

However, although I received sympathetic treatment from the gentleman concerned with our case, my visit made little difference. In view of the refusal of our neighbour to grant permission to the Electricity Board to cross his piece of land, certain prescribed paths would have to be followed, and as you can imagine, those paths would wend their way through skeins of red tape before arriving at a satisfactory conclusion.

We spent the weekend of the 19th July in Hove, relaxing for a change, before the impending move. We were to wake up early on Monday morning. Michael wanted to be in Guildford by eight a.m. to open the office, before driving me to the bungalow. We were ready to leave before seven o'clock and we switched on the television to see the first two men on the moon (Armstrong and Aldrin), eerily bouncing their way over its dusty surface.

Somehow, that historic event made our day seem all the more momentous and adventurous.

Coincidentally, Joan and Reg were moving too, to a house high up in the North Downs. Joan had three boys of school age, and ten years or so of her married life had been spent in that street. She was weeping as they drove away.

As for me, I shed not a tear as we drove off in the opposite direction. The house had served its purpose. It had acted as a sort of home for two and a half years, but I had sunk no roots there.

We arrived at the bungalow with the bulk of our furniture—our bed—on top of the van, and Michael immediately began work on the most important job of the day —the connecting of our gas stove, an elderly model, with only three legs. The important thing about it was that it was able to be connected to a bottle of gas. There was no gas laid on, so the cooker was something of a survival kit. Even the iron was to be heated upon it. Old-fashioned or not, together with packets of candles, boxes of matches and torch batteries, our three-legged friend was our sole means of providing heat, hot water and light (as well as cooking facilities for quite a long time to come.

With hindsight, we know there were things we could have done to make life a little easier. For example, we should have purchased a simple device which allows you to be connected to two bottles of gas and transfer from an empty one to a full one when necessary.

Without this facility, I lived constantly with the thrill—or fear—of running out of gas; and although we usually had spare bottles, I could neither lift them nor manoeuvre the spanner to connect them to the cooker.

It became a ritual to start the day, as we always had, by bathing. This involved heating three saucepans and a very large kettle on the cooker, and as soon as he had emptied his own water into the bath, Michael would fill up the receptacles for Robert or me. Sometimes I would bath Robert first, and then add a second helping of cooked water for myself. The little extra depth this provided gave me a feeling of luxury, though sometimes it had cooled so much, it was only equivalent to the cold water I would have added anyway. I was rather envious of Michael, as his large frame displaced so much water that he was actually covered by it, whilst I, at a little over half his thirteen stone, could never achieve that and had to be satisfied with sitting in a fairly deep puddle.

We continued this practice right through into the winter, when to start the day with a percentage of one's body preheated seemed like a good idea.

The main problem in July, however, was not lack of heat, but too much of it. We had no fridge, and the butter, the milk, and the meat had to be bought in the smallest possible quantities. Icecream, yoghurt and even frozen peas were a forgotten luxury, and the daily walk to the shops, carrying as much as possible on Robert's study pushchair, became another ritual.

I have never been much of a walker and in my mind I marked off the route into quarters. I had a choice between taking a narrow footpath which led away from the bungalow to the right towards the village, and ran behind half a dozen houses on the main road, or walking to the left along a pathway which connected with another wider lane and then to the main road. I was resentful of any extra steps, so I initially took the route to the right, since the footpath took perhaps five minutes off the journey time. Thick holly bushes grew up high on either side of the pathway, giving it a mysterious atmosphere that was not pleasant. As summer wore on, I felt rather like the Sleeping Beauty's prince fighting my way through the bushes. However, when they were trimmed, the sharp prickles covered the ground and made walking in open sandals almost an impossibility. I then took the alternative route, which eventually passed the houses whose gardens backed on to the footpath. I really preferred this route, as it meant that I occasionally saw human life and it was also easier for me to negotiate with the pushchair. The short cut joined the other road at an old fashioned 'kissing gate', and the end of the first quarter of my journey was marked by a brick wall on the outside of which was a rambling rose and a border of salvias. I thought it was very kind of the person who lived there to attend to these plants, when he couldn't see them himself from the inside of the wall.

The second stretch was the most boring, having only fields to observe, and this ended at the junction with another main road. A few houses appeared at this point, the main attraction of these being masses of rhododendron bushes that filled their gardens. I used to feast my eyes on the rich colours—the reds and purples and pinks—and hope that one day I might be able to offer these sights to a person passing my home.

Towards the end of the third leg of the journey was the petrol station, which seemed to me to mark the beginning of civilisation, and shortly after that came the whole range of shops, (all six of them) selling newspapers, groceries, hardware and meat, two public houses—and that was the beginning and end of the village.

Before we moved in, we had occasionally taken a Sunday afternoon stroll to the village just to get the 'feel' of the place, and it always seemed entirely deserted.

However, I soon found that during the week, it was a busy little place, where the many local car owners often chose to make their purchases, in preference to the bigger towns and shopping centres within a two to four mile radius. For the time being, I was without that choice, but I soon found the friendly shopkeepers preferable to the detached supermarket staff.

The village shopkeeper is 'owned' by the village; they know his business and he knows theirs. For me, suddenly and for the first time, totally in isolation, the friendly chat at the end of my half hour walk was a lifeline—my only link with humanity. The hubbub of our old office/home contrasted dramatically with our quiet bungalow, for as well as the other essentials that we lacked, we were also without car and telephone. Consequently, lines of communication with the outside world were cut off, and although there were six other houses in the vicinity of our land, I rarely saw any signs of life emanating from them. Our nearest neighbour had in fact been widowed during the period of our building, for we had met her and her husband once in the early days. Although I often saw her television flashing through the windows and heard her dogs yapping as I passed by, I did not feel able to inflict myself upon her.

Our other near neighbours, Doug and Beryl, in the foot of whose garden we resided, were almost invisible from autumn onwards. If only we had had a telephone, we, or they might have picked it up to say, 'Why don't you come over? Have a coffee—have a sherry,' but to walk to someone's front door to say the same is a much more difficult task. So we saw each other by chance, and infrequently.

Robert and I were now each other's main companions for the major part of the day. But in some ways, I felt like one of two incompatible prisoners, sharing the same cell. There was no contemporary or friend like Joan with whom he could stay for an hour or two, not even the facility of leaving him in the office with Michael, as I had done in the past. Robert was a sociable child, and possibly missing the activity of the office himself, constantly sought my presence. I, on the other hand, yearned for a period of complete solitude. Including him in the daily chores doubled or trebled the length of time they took, and I never found time to play with him. Sometimes I grumbled and told him to go away and play with his toys, but he still seemed to have no interest in doing so. Often in desperation, I would place him in his cot for an afternoon nap and sit reading, unkindly ignoring rising murmurs of complaint from an unsleepy child.

Another wedge between us was his masculinity. There had been a period when as a small baby, he had felt so much a part of me that I felt uneasy when I was away from him. Now he was no longer my baby, but a small boy who was inclined to be naughty or daring at times, and who had no wish to be frustrated in his desires by a mother saying, 'No.' As an only child myself, I was inexperienced at dealing with children, and having had mainly female cousins, I regarded small boys as an alien breed, and was often surprised, irritated or aggrieved by the very normal disobedience of a toddler. Without a companion of my own age, I was unable to share my child-rearing problems with anyone else. At the same time, I was aware that Robert's life, too, must have become more empty. Guiltily compensating for the unchanging and uneventful passage of each day, I would draw his attention to the arrival of a friendly robin, Max, the visiting dog who came to turn our dustbin over and collected a biscuit from Robert's tiny hand for his pains, or the magpies that swept dramatically across the garden.

I got quite fond of Max, the wandering labrador, like many lonely people who become attached to animals. I pictured him saving me in some dramatic situation and even considered writing this in the form of a short story. However, I was not sufficiently fired with enthusiasm to put pen to paper and, in any case, there never seemed to be quite time in the day for such pursuits.

By the end of the first six weeks of our 'no-mod-cons' existence, Michael had taken our old electric fridge (a silly piece of bachelor-size equipment), and by dint of some brilliant engineering, had converted it into a machine operated by bottled gas. Admittedly, it was highly inefficient, but it served our purpose, and enabled me to cut down a little on my journeys to and from the village.

Our first visitors, Ruth and Roger, had arrived within a month of our moving in. The bungalow was a great improvement on our first home, and despite its unfinished nature, I could show it with some pride to my friends.

Nevertheless, in the early weeks, we were not in the state of readiness I had hoped for. Very few of the furnishings were ready and worst of all, and despite my protestations, there was simply no floor covering in the major part of the house and we clattered around raising dust on the concrete floors.

But slowly things took shape; with the arrival of the furnishings, the lounge took on the elegant appearance I had pictured in my mind. The restful shades I had chosen became an extension of the colours of the countryside, and the curtains acted as a frame for the view outside, the five stately trees that were the focal point of our drive, backed by fields and with very little intrusion of houses into the landscape.

The arrival of the carpet also enabled me to demote our old living room carpet to our bedroom. Although it didn't fit awfully well, I managed to get the worst bits under the bed, so that at least our feet came in contact with a warm surface instead of the cold concrete. It stayed there until the early seventies, but by that time I had become accustomed and unsurprised at our slow progress, and even rather appreciated it, for each innovation could be enjoyed on its own account.

At the present time, however, we did not even run a car and Michael frequently travelled the four miles to the office by bus. We had owned a rather smart second hand Wolseley, which we had abandoned at the 'site' when it developed a major fault. To our shame, it had remained there, gradually decaying for the next few years. Therefore the event which ought to have made a lot of difference to me, the passing of my driving test in

August, made no difference at all. Since I was quite petrified at the idea of driving on my own, I was really quite relieved that no car, other than the untaxed, uninsured Wolseley, sat outside the door waiting for me to jump into it.

It was still good walking weather, and the summer sunshine stretched on into the autumn.

I, who had never appreciated the delights of the countryside before, now gazed out of my windows at unbearably beautiful scenes. The majestic oaks, acacias and chestnuts at the front of the house retained their stately dignity at each change of season, and even though the view from my kitchen window was marred by the weedridden wilderness that was our own garden, the boundary was marked by two copper beeches and an enormous conifer, perhaps sixty feet high, as well as the more commonplace deciduous trees. The giant conifer would remain—a symbol of life in the depths of winter—but the copper beeches would first turn scarlet at their climax, before the brilliant foliage finally withered and died.

Now the mornings were sometimes cool before the sun emerged; then Robert and I would wander outdoors, crunching leaves and twigs beneath our feet as we collected dead sticks to make up a fire. The hedgerows were full of blackberries and we picked out the biggest and best on our walks to and from the village.

But we still felt strangers in this countrified world, Robert and I. He would not set foot outside the door without me; and I for my part, felt unnatural carrying out these rural tasks. I was at loss in this unpeopled world. The beauty of the surroundings did not make up for the lack of humankind. Sometimes, as I gazed at the view, I longed for a car to appear, spilling out friends to share it with me.

My old friend Susan, who would now have lived so close to me, had moved to her native Ireland with her husband, Bruce and her two children. However, her English parents-in-law lived a mere mile from my home, and one day a car did indeed draw up unexpectedly and Susan and her family emerged.

It was a wonderful surprise, although the house was not in a state of tidiness I would have liked; the hearth was not swept, and Robert had been sitting in his high chair aiming bread fingers at the still un-linoed kitchen floor. But no-one had ever arrived on days when I had been efficient—and actually, they still never do.

Susan's visit gave me the opportunity to invite her for dinner—and it was one of the few occasions of its kind that autumn, for only special friends were invited to share our hardships. Candle-lighting time had gradually been brought forward to the early evening, and the room looked at its best, decked with candles and illuminated too by the blazing log fire.

We had ordered a lorry load of logs from a local man, and each day, I would clean out the grate and relay the fire; first the paper, then the kindling wood, finally one or two of the logs. I became quite an expert; for although the days were delightful, as darkness fell, the house became chilly and the roaring fire became a necessity, not just an attractive feature of our lounge.

Bruce warned me: 'Collect plenty of timber now, while it's dry.'

He was right, of course; the fire was one of the mainstays of our existence. I didn't like to think too far ahead of the approaching winter, but we couldn't expect this golden Indian summer to last much longer.

It was Robert's birthday in October, his second birthday, on which another child should have been born; but I had no feelings of regret about that now. How could we have introduced another baby into this situation without proper heating or washing facilities? As it was, we had to make a regular weekend trip to the launderette in one of the firm's vans, packed out with washing. However, we were thinking again about another pregnancy; I wanted Robert to have a companion, while he was young enough to enjoy a brother or sister. Perhaps a two year age difference was a little narrow, bearing in mind the apparent contrariness of two-year-olds, but a gap of another six months—that surely must be ideal. I did not imagine that Fate would play any more unkind tricks on me.

I had, for some time, been summoning up my courage to invite Michael's family over; we had always invited them in appropriate sections before. But now the bungalow was big enough to house all of them on one occasion, and a birthday seemed an auspicious enough occasion to entertain Robert's aunts, uncles and grandma. Including ourselves, the family amounted to nine adults and four 'halves'. The question was, could I cope with the sheer numerical impact of Michael's exuberant (and efficient) family?

It was the chip on my shoulder about being less efficient than my sisters-in-law that made me accept the challenge. There was always the chance that with our present difficulties, I might show up to better advantage.

So I roasted and baked and fried; and dusted and 'carpet-swept'. (I couldn't use my vacuum cleaner, of course.) Robert's birthday—and the family—arrived on a perfect autumn day. We had homemade cakes for tea; then in a Luben-like frenzy, they rushed outside to find conkers and they played enthusiastically with one-ers and two-ers, dropping chestnut shells on the carpet; but never mind, it had looked fine when they arrived, and that was the important thing. As dusk fell, we lit the candles and unveiled the buffet supper on a long trestle table in the wide hall. Cold chicken and roast beef, cold fried fish, cooked in the Jewish style; carefully prepared vegetable salad, potato salad, tomato salad; and fresh fruit (with cream for those errant members of the family who would flout the Jewish tradition not to combine milk with meat). I had made a success of it and I knew it; and it was difficult not to glow with pride in the warmth of the fire and the appreciation.

As always I felt how good it was to be part of a family, and how lucky I was to have acquired this good-humoured bunch of brothers and sisters.

Another member of the family, Michael's first cousin Colin, a wizard with motors, was an occasional visitor. At that time, although not living in the vicinity, he worked for the local A.A. and made a point of dropping in spontaneously.

Once he called in when I had run out of gas and drove me to the local suppliers to buy a gas bottle and connected it himself.

53

On another occasion, he actually let me drive his own car into the village to get some shopping.

Apart from purely sociable reasons for calling, he was interested in our old Wolseley and spent a lot of time renovating the engine. He was a meticulous worker and Michael also asked him to look at the generator which we had been given by a scrap dealer.

He was quite content to spend hours working outside and whenever I asked what he was doing he always seemed to be 'cleaning the carbon brushes.'

Sometimes he shared with us a candlelit dinner, and it was always a pleasure to have a guest at our table. But these few social occasions were merely oases in a desert of unrelieved difficulties, and as we moved towards winter, it was difficult to quell my increasing frustration and loneliness.

No Electricity, No Heat, No Car, No Phone,
November ...*with apologies to Thomas Hood*

The days grew shorter and colder and the tensions increased. We awoke in darkness and breakfasted by candlelight. Last night's dinner plates and greasy pots and pans awaited my attention in daylight.

Now, though I lit the fire early each chill morning, the house temperature would not reach 60°F. until around midday. At the first glimmer of autumn sunshine, I would open the windows to induce some warmth into the house. But it was a vain effort.

Water streamed down the windows daily and each morning the bedspread was wet with condensation like a dew-soaked lawn.

Many times, the heavy use of gas in the morning caused the bottle to run out after Michael had left the house. Then Robert and I would walk the mile to the telephone to contact him, only to be confronted on many occasions by the answering machine. On those days, I could only boil a kettle on the fire for tea, or cook a tin of soup. Spiders' webs bejewelled with misty drops were draped across each holly bush, as we set out on our expeditions. I observed them, but was too irritated by the chilly and too often abortive treks to appreciate Nature's artistry.

We were no longer playing an amusing game. I had always disliked darkness; now I often returned from our shopping expeditions in dusk, gazing with envy at the brightly lit homes I passed. Filled with despondency, I would fumble around for matches. The daylight hours were not long enough for everything I had to do. Often I was forced to go out into the thick blackness of the night to get in more logs to keep the fire going, accompanied only by the small circle of light from the torch. Michael often brought in a basketful of logs, but he worked long and late hours, and the possibility of the fire going out merely because of his absence was unthinkable.

To a certain extent, Michael was insulated from the problem.

When he came home in the evening, he would sit in the lounge-cum-dining room where the fire was burning brightly and the drawn curtains kept the room at a comfortable and pleasant temperature. Weekends were often spent escaping to other members of the family. In any case, Michael was a warm person, often not noticing the cold at all, whilst I was acutely aware of it. I felt therefore that this was my personal martyrdom, and when I described it to my friends, made sure they realised how long-suffering I was.

Why didn't we give in? We had always doubted that the Electricity Board would accept money from us, but we could have contacted the Colonel privately; and in our reluctance to do this there was an element of pride and an unwillingness to be manipulated, feelings shared by both of us. In any case, initially we were under the impression that the Electricity Board's compulsory powers would be implemented much more quickly, and had not really imagined that we would still be without electricity in the winter. Even now, it was difficult to believe that the Electricity Board would allow this situation to continue for much longer. There was the financial aspect too; we were always short of money, but in my heart, I do not think this was the main reason for digging our heels in.

However, Michael was not insensitive to the increasing difficulties and when he came home one evening to find me warming frozen fingers in front of the fire, before returning to the kitchen to peel potatoes, he said, 'We can't go on like this.'

Within a day or so, he made two purchases—an oil heater and a gas light—and of the two, it was the latter which was the most spirit lifting.

With a young child in the house, we had not previously given much thought to an oil heater. Now we lifted the carpet, and for safety's sake, screwed the heater down to the concrete. Thereafter, we had a delivery of paraffin each week, and ran the heater night and day, but to be honest, the difference in temperature was not great.

The light had much more impact! We attached it by a long flex to a smallish gas bottle, which was not too heavy, and transported it between the kitchen and lounge. It was almost as good as a light bulb; miracle of miracles, almost possible to read by it. How wonderful it was to come in from the dark outside and not be faced with the prospect of lighting seven or eight candles and balancing them on saucers. How satisfying to light the delicate gas mantle and see the little flame turn into a bright glow. And how heartbreaking when, in our eagerness to light it or replace the mantle, we accidently destroyed it with clumsy fingers, when we had no replacement. But we soon learned to avoid such disasters.

'One day,' Michael promised extravagantly, 'I'll turn this place into a palace of lights.'

Buoyed up by the morale-boosting effect of the latest purchases, I asked my two aunts from Hove to stay for a weekend. It was a fairly foolish thing to do, but on the one hand, I wanted to invite people to share our lonely adventure, and at the same time I wanted to behave as normally as possible. Social occasions were small goals to aim for. The days seemed less monotonous with the prospect of visitors ahead and there seemed to be a purpose in boring domestic chores.

The Aunties were my closest relations with the exception of my parents, and I wanted the chance to show off to them my improving skills in cooking and running our attractive new home. My father was a sick man, and it was quite impossible to subject him to our problems. The Aunties, however, were a pair of sports and, despite the fact that Auntie Betty was over sixty and Auntie Ethel was approaching it, I felt that they would put up with our difficulties without complaint.

Unfortunately, in one respect, the Aunties' visit was something of a disaster, for as soon as we had crossed the South Downs in the car we had hired to transport them, we discovered that the rest of the South was covered in snow, which grew worse as we drove towards Surrey. Only Michael's quick reactions prevented us from being stuck on any of the hillier roads that had entrapped other motorists who had attempted them, but the journey was long and slow, and the bungalow only a few degrees above freezing when we arrived home. We would not have chosen to inflict such conditions on the Aunties, but they endured them stoically and merely congratulated themselves on remembering their hot water bottles.

They came from the generation that lived through the Blitz and they had done war work together in the sugar beet factories of Lincolnshire. This small adventure would simply add another tale to their repertoire.

The next day, the sun melted the snow and shone through the windows. We looked out and admired the chaffinches and bullfinches, swaying to and fro on the long, long grass in the garden. Perhaps we were not quite mad to live here.

The first snow dispelled any doubts we might have had that winter would finally arrive. But we had been lucky; we had had a wonderful summer, and a bright and beautiful autumn. It could have been so much worse.

Our next visitors were cousin Colin's sister and fiancé and in their honour, we were able to provide lights in the lounge for one hour.

Colin's occasional visits and careful work on the generator had eventually borne fruit, for we were finally able to connect it up. However, we had lost touch with the electrician who had carried out the first stage of wiring a year before, and wires stuck out of the walls, awaiting the fixing of switches and points, which Michael had not yet found the time to do.

When the generator was finally ready, Michael sent me out for light fittings for the lounge, and the first connections were made. However, we could only afford to have lighting on special occasions, for the generator used a gallon of petrol in an hour, and even if it had provided lights for the whole house, it would still have been too costly to run on a regular basis. In addition, the ancient contraption made a noise like a steam engine and emitted dreadful fumes from its exhaust, which we aimed in the direction of the Colonel's empty field, next to us.

Disappointment that the generator could not be the means of solving all our problems was slightly mitigated by the resolution of another difficulty. We were going to have a telephone.

We had always assumed that our principled Colonel had

prevented us from having this facility, since its wires would have to cross his footpath. However, in the course of a general enquiry, which Michael made from the office, he discovered that we had misjudged him; for it was our near neighbour, Mrs Baker, who had failed to sign the forms agreeing to our telephone wire being linked to hers, at a point near the eaves of her house.

'Oh, if only we'd known,' I moaned, thinking of the many unnecessary walks to the village, just to use the phone. I felt sure that Mrs Baker's action, or rather, lack of it, had been one of simple forgetfulness rather than deliberate awkwardness.

My initial visit confirmed that she was completely co-operative. She would be happy to sign the appropriate form.

'But you'll have to hurry,' she told me; 'I shall be moving at the end of the week.' It appeared that she had not been happy there since her husband's death and was returning to South Africa. The house had been sold to a young couple. It was quite a thrilling thought for me that our near neighbours would be contemporaries and perhaps 'kindred spirits'.

Without delay, I returned to Mrs Baker with the required form, and a few days later, I was at the house yet again to make overtures of friendship to the new occupant.

I had to summon up a lot of courage to do that for I'm not normally a very outgoing sort of person; I really prefer friendships handed to me on a plate. Nevertheless, I had reached desperation level, and was prepared to go to new lengths.

The girl who answered the door was dressed in a bright red dressing gown. I had become quite used to getting up early and was quite smug to find someone with my old bad habits. I introduced myself and invited her to join me for coffee during the course of the morning. She was not very responsive, but she agreed.

As pleased as if I was preparing for a date with a male, I rushed home and tidied up; prepared the fire, put the milk on for coffee. But she didn't come—not on that or any other morning. It was a blow—to my pride as much as anything else, for it seemed that a young woman of my own age had summed me up in less than five minutes and decided that my company was not worth having.

Much later, when I discovered that she was a 'Bunny girl', living with the young man in residence, I appreciated that she probably had such a totally different life style from my own, that it would have been difficult for us to find anything in common. Realising that, did much to repair my damaged pride, though not my disappointment at the lack of a companion near at hand.

However, on the same morning as the coffee non-event, telephone engineers arrived and connected up the wires to our house. A vast telephone pole became the corner post of our land, blending surprisingly well with the trees. Only a few days more and our period of total isolation was ended; once more we were in touch with the world.

There is a limit to how long a man running a business can do so without his own vehicle. Despite our shame at the decaying Wolseley adorning one corner of our 'garden' and despite the more or less unchanged financial problems, Michael decided to buy a new car—a new old car, I should say—and one night, a roomy Consul arrived and on exchange of a hundred pounds or so, became ours.

That very evening, Michael took us out for a trial run and the car proved satisfactory. On the way back, he pointed out the soakaway, running alongside the holly hedge that formed the boundary between the main lane and an adjacent garden.

'Whatever you do,' he warned, 'Don't go down that ditch.'

Indignantly I replied that I wasn't quite such a fool as that. The ditch was so obvious; I couldn't understand why he should bother to mention it.

Since the car was not to be used exclusively by Michael, but would be left with me occasionally so that I could build up some confidence, Michael rang our insurance brokers the next day.

'You can take the car to the top of the lane,' he told me later. 'But don't go on the main road. You'll have insurance cover tomorrow, but until then you can only drive on the lane, because it's private land.'

Michael could see no reason for me to delay taking a first experimental run in the car, though I would have waited quite happily till the following day.

Even for me, however, there was not too much difficulty in this short run. Along our slightly bumpy lane; then right turn and down the lane leading to the main road. One or two hundred yards of straight forward driving and that was the full extent of the trip. But now that I was at the main road—what should I do to get back again? I wasn't very good at reversing straight backwards, so the answer seemed to be a three-point turn. I didn't like the idea of reversing into the wood—I might hit a small tree or find it too bumpy, so I carefully reversed to the right on to the grassy bank in front of the holly hedge. Too late, I remembered the soakaway. I stopped quickly and tried to pull forward; I thought I had stopped in ample time, but my judgement was poor; when I got out of the car to investigate, I saw to my horror that the car's back wheels were half way down the ditch.

A small elderly gentleman, white-haired and rosy-faced, appeared on the scene. I vaguely recognised him as a local 'walker'. It would probably make his day to become a knight in shining armour and rescue a damsel in distress. I didn't want to hurt his feelings by telling him that my husband was within striking distance. In addition, if I could have extricated myself from the situation without telling Michael what had happened, I would have done so happily. I let my would-be rescuer potter about the wood for a few minutes, looking for bricks to put in front of the tyres, but with the wheels spinning each time I tried to pull forward, I knew our feeble efforts were to no avail and I told the elderly gentleman that I would have to fetch my husband.

I hardly dared look at Michael's face when I told him the news, and I stayed at home while he angrily stomped off to examine my handiwork.

Thank goodness, we had a regular delivery of bread. Just at

the right moment, the breadman arrived in his van and towed us out of trouble. In fact the aftermath of comments from Michael was probably worse than the incident. He just didn't seem to realise that there's a world of difference between driving down a ditch and *reversing* down a ditch.

Let There be Light

It was about the middle of December when we received the letter.

It was from the Colonel; he had written to the Electricity Board saying that he was prepared to accept a lesser sum as compensation from them, as he 'did not like to think of the Lubens being without electricity for Christmas'.

Was he genuine? I couldn't decide. I had often seen him driving around when I was walking with Robert. He never looked at me; I believe he couldn't look me in the face.

On the other hand, he may just have realised that the powers of the Electricity Board would catch up with him soon, and he might as well try to compromise.

'Let's send them a cheque for the balance,' I said to Michael. There were at least three months of winter still to come and I was suddenly aware that I couldn't go on much longer.

We sent a cheque to the Electricity Board right away, but within a few days it was back. They were prepared to agree to the Colonel's suggestion and since they were settling the matter themselves, they would not require our money.

The New Year, 1970, was only a fortnight away, and suddenly it had a magic sound to it.

We had arranged to go to a dinner dance in a hotel on New Year's Eve with the family, and I was looking forward to it tremendously. We hadn't been out for such a long time, other than family visits.

'It's going to be a good year, Michael,' I kept telling him. 'We've got the telephone; we're going to get electricity—and a new baby in the summer. I just know it's going to be a good year.'

We hadn't told many people about the baby this time. As in my first two pregnancies, there were no obvious signs yet—no appreciable weight gain, no swelling of the limbs, no nausea. I was lucky; I felt extremely fit. But it was difficult to be extra careful when I felt so normal.

Michael had recommenced the task of connecting up the electricity, for we had never located our original electrician. Except for the lounge, a whole houseful of wires stuck out of the walls or hung from the ceiling in clusters, and each one must be followed from its source to its eventual outcome.

It crossed my mind briefly, when I was helping Michael identify the electric wires, that some people said that stretching upwards wasn't a very good idea. So I tried to be careful and used my kitchen stool, when it was necessary to reach up to the ceiling.

At intervals, I would hear banging from the loft above.

'Can you hear me? Do you know where I am?'

'You're in Robert's bedroom, (kitchen/bathroom, etc.).'

'Can you see the wires hanging from the ceiling? Take hold of one and tie a knot in it.'

All the wires eventually had knots or S-bends or just came straight down and that all apparently had some meaning for Michael, and was carefully noted on a complex wiring diagram.

It was such a painstaking job; it was heartbreaking to think that the electric power would be sitting outside our house, ready and waiting for us before we were ready to receive it.

A few days before Christmas, a group of navvies arrived and in Arctic conditions, dug a trench the length of the lane. As snow descended from the bleak heavens, I thought of offering them all some whisky; but I always felt uncomfortable making such grand gestures, and in the end, my nerve failed me. They were probably warmer than I was anyway.

The Christmas holiday was to be spent partly with Michael's mother and partly with my parents in Hove. Michael could do very little of the electrical work before we left home. The lounge, of course, was now equipped with light and, in addition, an electric fire and television. Without an aerial, the flickering picture from the T.V. must have resembled the early moving pictures, but after such a long period without that form of escapism in the home, we were satisfied—possibly even as enthusiastic as the viewers of the early movies.

But for now, the escape was to the warmer climes of our parents' homes. I had packaged the children's presents and I had sent Christmas cards to all my non-Jewish friends, including one to the Colonel, which I inscribed 'With many thanks for your kind gesture'. This was hardly a kind gesture of my own—rather I had some feeling of rubbing salt into the wound of his shame, if indeed it did exist.

With a clear conscience and with a feeling of relief, we abandoned our house and our problems to enjoy the family holiday, but at the end of four days, we reluctantly prepared to return.

I noticed that there was a musical on the television which I wanted to see and tried to convince myself that that was a genuine inducement to return home early in the evening.

'Let's hurry,' I told Michael, 'so that we can get home in time to watch "Carousel".'

So hurry we did; the car zoomed up and down the South and North Downs (on this occasion there was no snow) and swerved round the bends. I didn't really mind Michael driving fast, but by the time we arrived home, I felt slightly travel-sick. There was also an ominous ache at the pit of my stomach.

I tried to ignore it, as I sat a foot or so away from the electric fire, failing to absorb any warmth from it at all, watching the fluttering screen with no real enthusiasm.

But the dull ache did not go and eventually although it was nearing ten o'clock, I was forced to telephone the doctor.

The answer was predictable. 'Go to bed; rest. Ring the doctor in the morning if there are still problems.'

For nearly a week I lay in bed.

One of the local team of doctors, a pleasant Scottish woman called to see me.

'How many times is this going to happen?' I asked, unreasonably angry. 'Must I just lie and wait for a miscarriage to happen?'

She assured me that if I were to miscarry this time, something would be done to help me next time. One miscarriage could be Nature's method of removing a malformed child. Two suggested a pattern where the mother might have a weakness.

My mother, after all, had had five miscarriages before I was born, and it was probably the fear of following in her footsteps that had caused me to want our first child so early in our marriage.

But in spite of the doctor's reassurance about the future, I was filled with indignation and disbelief that such a thing could be allowed to happen to me twice, and that those around me were apparently powerless to do anything positive to prevent it, other than to recommend that I should stay in bed and rest. Never before had I considered what a spirit of optimism my mother must have had to have weathered this demoralising experience five times.

Endeavouring to help on a practical level, the doctor asked if there was somewhere Robert could stay, so that I could rest. Michael and I, who had not previously considered sending Robert away, mulled over the problem and agreed that it would be a good idea. We decided that he would be happiest with my sister-in-law Sonia. Sonia adored children and her own boy, Stephen was old enough at eight to allow her to devote a little extra time to Robert.

'You won't mind going to Auntie Sonia?' I asked him and solemnly he replied that he would not. I tried to explain the situation to him in simple terms. I hoped that this time he would be better prepared for his parting from me.

Luckily, Sonia was entirely happy to take Robert and without much delay, Michael transported him to her home in Epsom.

On the second day, there was an office panic—a pressing call. Michael had to leave me alone; we rang my mother and asked if she could stay with me. She could stay for one day, she said, and arrived by train, bearing food— as mothers do; a rosy-cheeked, brown-haired capable woman in her late sixties, her looks belying her age. How could she stay any longer, she said, there was Daddy to look after. I realised her role had changed; her priority now was her sick husband, not her child. Not for the first time did I regret the passing of the days when I was tucked into bed and cosseted by my warmhearted mother. But I was a married woman now; and the apron strings should have been severed a long time ago.

Having spent most of the day in bed, I came into the lounge and lay with my feet up on the settee in front of the log fire, covered with blankets. Towards the end of the day, my mother left me to catch her train home, and before Michael returned that night, I watched the traditional celebrations of Hogmanay on the inadequate television. As far as I was concerned, 1970 came in, not with a bang, but with a whimper of self pity on my lips.

'And I thought it was going to be such a great year!'

But I had not lost heart entirely and when Ruth telephoned a day or so later, her words filled me with a ridiculous hope.

She had hoped to call in; she and Roger were going to be in the area. I would have loved to have seen her, but I told her the present situation—then she told me her news— she was expecting a baby at the end of July. I was convinced then, quite irrationally, that I would not miscarry—that it was fated that our second children would be born at around the same time, just as Robert and Lawrence had been.

As the week wore on, little changed. I lay in our lilac-coloured bedroom with the radio as my companion, watching squirrels, silhouetted against the matt white sky, playing on the naked branches of the trees.

Michael was to be seen periodically with screwdriver, switch, plug or wire in his hands, reporting to me, 'I've done the kitchen/hall/bedroom' and so on.

Without pain, and with only a small loss of blood, I began to feel adventurous. Towards the end of the week, I got up once or twice to prepare meals for us. It's impossible to ask a woman to stay in bed indefinitely, particularly if she is unsupervised.

The climax came one morning. I awoke to find myself haemorrhaging. And with the haemorrhage, came recognisable regular contractions, just as if I was in labour. To the layman who does not know how much blood her body is meant to lose, there is nothing so frightening as the feeling that she is going to bleed to death. The doctor, with his superior knowledge knows that the sufferer can certainly hold on till the end of morning surgery, and no amount of panic-stricken calls will shake his faith. Despite my previous experience, I was no less fearful on this occasion.

Eventually, however, the doctor arrived and promptly rang for an ambulance to transport me to hospital. This time, I made sure my suitcase was adequately packed.

The houseman arrived at my bedside without his bedside manner.

'Rustle me up some scrambled eggs,' he shouted to the staff nurse. 'I haven't had any lunch.' He examined me, glaring as though it was my fault. Perhaps he thought I'd done it deliberately.

A red spot on his cuff contrasted with its otherwise immaculate whiteness.

'You've got blood on your sleeve,' I told him maliciously. My blood!

I was surprised that they didn't rush me off to the theatre, as they had done before. This time a nurse arrived with a saline drip.

'What's that for?' I asked, surprised.

'Oh, just in case we have to give you any blood. We're going to keep you on bed rest for a little while.'

My heart leapt at the words 'bed rest'. There was a chance that they were going to save the baby. A simple urine test apparently confirmed the possibility that I could still be pregnant. My hopes, which had been dashed by the explosion of blood from my body, were raised once again.

Hitched up to the saline drip, I became a virtual prisoner. I was aware that my left arm did not contain a good vein, so I was not surprised that the drip was attached to my right arm. This was strapped to a foot long splint, which happened to be the only one they could find.

Thus I was incapacitated by my immovable right hand and my inefficient left hand, and forbidden even to sit up, so that at meal times a young nurse had to feed me in a semi-supine position. There is a limit to the amount of cosseting that even I find acceptable.

I put up a bit of a fight when it came to bedpans, and they were kind enough to bring me a commode, for which little dignity I was most grateful.

I had little discomfort and I refused a sleeping pill, but when night fell, I was restless; my stomach seemed to be heaving about. A nurse bent over my bed.

'Can't you sleep?' she asked.

'Perhaps I should have taken a pill,' I replied. Then I confided: 'I keep thinking I can feel the baby moving.'

She seemed to shudder.

'Oh, how awful,' she said. She didn't seem to understand.

'Perhaps the baby's all right,' I explained to her. 'Please tell someone, so they won't take it away.'

She went away; I heard her talking to another woman. I heard the reply echoing back from the quiet corridor.

'Absolute rubbish! She can't feel the baby yet.'

I wanted to explain to them that perhaps my dates were wrong. Perhaps I was sixteen weeks pregnant, not twelve weeks.

The young nurse came back with a sleeping pill, and I settled down to sleep.

In the course of the next couple of days I acquired a new neighbour, a young woman who was also in danger of miscarrying for the second time, and who, like me, had one child already.

We compared notes and it was amazing to discover that we had experienced the same emotions—the same feelings of guilt, of inadequacy as well as anger and sorrow. Marooned, as we were in our beds, we had nothing to do but rest and talk, and for those few days, we became as sisters in the sharing of our mutual experience.

One morning the consultant arrived, with his respectful entourage in attendance. Unsmiling, he conducted his examination. Immediately afterwards, he informed his staff he would carry out a 'D&C'.

Flabbergasted, I protested stutteringly and inarticulately.

'But what about the pregnancy tests—they were positive? I felt the baby moving!'

'I am sure the foetus has broken up during the haemorrhage,' he replied unemotionally.

As a parting shot, he ordered: 'She's very constipated; give her an enema before the operation.'

They left me in the curtained off cubicle. I was glad they had not opened the curtains, because now that I was alone, the tears poured from me. Why had they allowed me to believe the baby might be saved? Why had they given me extra care for two days only now to rob me of my child? Why had they not taken it away the first moment I entered the hospital?

My tears spent, I waited patiently while a middle-aged nurse fumblingly tried to administer an enema. She had to get help from some other nurses, and after their eventual success, I was reduced to an exhausted, limp rag. I half wondered if the doctor had only specified it to knock all the fight out of me, and indeed with the administration of the injection, I lay there unresisting and uncaring, as I was wheeled to the operating theatre.

The familiar tableau of green-overalled, masked figures met my eyes.

From a long way away, a voice asked, 'Have you any children?'

'Yes, a boy of two.'

The gap was widening; I had wanted a two year gap between my children, and now I would have to wait another year.

I drifted away into sleep.

When I awoke, I found I was no longer attached to the drip and I was allowed to sit up for the first time. As soon as the haziness of anaesthesia had left me, I conducted an animated conversation with my neighbour, which went on into the night. From the far corner of the ward came the shout: 'Aren't you two ever going to get to sleep?' and I was reminded that the bulk of my fellows in the ward were recovering from major surgery, whilst I was practically fit. The removal of my potential blood supply served to underline my now even less important status in the ranks of the sick.

By the next morning, I discovered that I would be discharged in twenty four hours, and after the more intensive care of the first couple of days, my speedy dispatch from hospital was an anticlimax. No guidance, no advice—just an appointment with Outpatients in six weeks' time, and out into the world.

I was no more than a body, whose parts had not been working properly. Like garage mechanics, they would put me back in working order and send me home. After all, what car ever receives an explanation from the repair man?

The anger I felt after this miscarriage lasted quite a long time. Apart from the self-directed anger at my own possible lack of sufficient caution, I felt I had been very badly treated by the hospital. For a while I half believed that they had robbed me of a living child, but even after I had returned to sanity, and doubted not that their physical treatment of me had been impeccable, I could see no reason why they should have allowed my hopes to be raised, causing me so much more distress than I had experienced during my first miscarriage.

Even if the consultant, presumably the decision maker, could not see me until a particular day, an explanation—a warning—given by the sister or staff nurse might have been a little help.

I had given up expecting the right sort of reactions from Michael. It was obviously a blind spot in his make-up. But I expected better understanding from the medical profession. They did not provide it whilst I was in hospital, and they did not provide it when I got home, neither after this nor my first miscarriage.

One day I was a pregnant woman, receiving the maximum care and attention. The next day I was an unpregnant woman receiving no automatic care, whatsoever. For the next six weeks, I would be regarded as a fit person, and no health visitor or other medical official would darken my door to determine whether I needed any help on an emotional level. The woman who has lost her baby has already received a blow undermining her confidence. She believes herself to be inadequate, and she believes her husband feels the same way, and quite possibly he does.

At this low point in her life, she is dropped by the Health Service, to the extent of removing her right to free prescriptions from the very day she leaves hospital. To a woman potentially at the edge of depression, this is a negation of her worth as a woman.

Luckily, I did not at any time reach the state medically known as depression. Of course I got depressed and disappointed, and I got angry, but, perhaps because I was aware of these emotions, I was not overwhelmed by them at any time. Once again I was told not to try to have another baby too soon; we had waited for about five months after the first miscarriage, and even that had apparently been too soon. Once again I faced that longing to be pregnant again—not even to have a baby— just to be in that blissful state of carrying around a wonderful secret— but this time I knew that the longing would fade in time and take on manageable proportions.

And anyway, there was the advent of electricity in our home, which despite all, could not be belittled.

There was also a bout of 'flu which struck us down, one by one, starting with Michael, who was almost as bad a patient as he was a nurse. None of us had been ill for ages; in fact it was quite remarkable how fit we had remained during the entire period when we had virtually no heat in the house—until now when comfort and warmth were returning.

Funny how I always thought that our house would be turned on magically, like Blackpool illuminations, and instead, it was a light bulb here and a power point there. Even on the very day when one of the powers-that-be from the Electricity Board came to check the completed work, Michael was working at fever pitch to get everything ready. And even after his work had been passed, there were sealed up wires tucked away in cupboards, waiting for the day when a surfeit of energy on Michael's part would cause them to be connected and the opening of a cupboard would automatically switch on a light within.

The very first circuit that Michael had tackled had included the immersion heater and what bliss it was to sink into a hot water bath without the prior water-boiling preparations.

One of the last connections was the electrical aspect of our oil-fired boiler. It was interesting to realise that the passable heating system in our old home, fired by an old fashioned oil burner, could have worked without electricity, (requiring only the lighting of a wick with a match) whilst our new automated one could not. It left us with a distinct feeling that we should not put ourselves totally at the mercy of automation. We had already demonstrated the value of an open fire and chimney, at a time when many people were boarding up their chimneys, and new homes were being built without them. Now, having learned to live with bottled gas, we retained our three-legged gas cooker while we gave a good deal of thought to our next step.

It was the middle of January when the lights went on, and despite the miscarriage, 1970 began to look pretty good from then on.

I and the Infernal Combustion Engine, etc.

It was so luxurious to have light and warmth once again, and now that we were actually living like a normal family, I invited everyone we knew to visit us. From March through to December, almost every weekend seemed to be occupied by someone coming to us or vice versa. My cousins came for the first time, and the brothers and sisters came in turn and even stayed the night. Lots of our friends visited us too; everyone was subjected to a healthy march over the large area of common and woodland which we treated as our country estate. They all had a tour of inspection of the house too and now that my faith in impossibilities really happening was restored, we blithely showed them the hole where the swimming pool would be, the gap where the built-in oven would be built in, the bare bathroom wall, and the roll of wallpaper that would in due course be stuck to it, Uncynically, we almost believed that they could see the finished picture that we could visualise in our mind's eye.

I visited the hospital and after a cursory examination, was dismissed with the usual statistics that two in five pregnancies or was it one in four spontaneously terminated. My visit to my G. P. was much more satisfying; first he reassured me about the bumpy ride from Brighton.

'If it hadn't been that, it would have been something else,' he told me, suggesting one or two other innocent pursuits that might have caused it just as easily.

And looking back, it is difficult to see why I felt quite so guilty, for if every woman could expect to miscarry as a result of the things I had done, there would be hordes of women taking fast car journeys and lifting heavy objects, instead of taking the proverbial hot bath and bottle of gin, or indeed instead of queuing up for abortions.

My main concern now, however, was the next pregnancy.

'As soon as you know you are pregnant,' he said. 'Come and see me. We will help you through it from the beginning.'

After that I put it out of my mind, knowing I must now wait, and when Ruth and Roger arrived for a weekend, with Ruth well into the middle of her pregnancy, I do not believe I felt too many pangs of jealousy.

The other all important event in January was the sale of our old home and office, and despite the great relief both to us and the Bank Manager, this was something of an anticlimax to me, since I was hardly involved in it. As a result of the sale, Michael now spent quite a lot of time at home, although he was looking around for a small lock-up office.

With the house now in some semblance of order, I felt able to invite my parents to stay and we chose a sunny weekend in June, when the countryside would be at its most pleasant. My timing proved to be faulty, for only a few days before the Visit, the washing machine went wrong and when they arrived, we were once again living on naked concrete floors.

I was accustomed to the washing machine being a little temperamental, and how much this was to do with having to wash Michael's entire rugby kit, including his boots, in bygone days, I never really knew. Every now and then, it would literally blow its top and emit froth and water in a thin stream. All that was needed was a speedy twiddle of knobs and sanity would usually be restored, and mopping up operations could be commenced.

On this occasion, I was following my normal routine, or lack of it (for things hadn't changed dramatically in three years of married life when I became aware that the machine was still filling with water, when I should have expected it to have stopped. Rushing to do the necessary twiddle, I found indeed that there was a shallow puddle forming on the kitchen floor. Going into action with squeezy mop and bucket, I soon noticed that the volume of water on the floor was increasing despite my efforts. This was an unexpected development, so I turned the washing machine off completely.

I had been working for a full ten minutes on swabbing the

decks, when I realised that the noise that kept on and on in my ears was the sound of the mains water running and running, and it came to me that for reasons best known to itself, the washing machine had continued to fill and spill throughout the entire floor washing session. I rushed to turn off the mains, and even as I did so, saw the dark stain of water spreading insidiously over half the hall carpet.

No time for independence or emancipation now. The important question was 'Where's Michael?'

A few phone calls to likely places unearthed a couple of the plumbers; they came over to see if they could help, but by that time, most of the water had been cleared up, leaving only a damp and soggy carpet, and...

One other thing which I didn't discover until I tried to boil a kettle for tea, for plumbers are great tea drinkers. A fault on the wiring under the concrete kitchen floor which operated all electricity in the kitchen, lounge and boiler room. No electricity—Again!

But Michael was not defeated, though he found me quite hysterical on the subject, when he finally arrived home. A few electrical miracles were performed and then he was able to find the time to say to me, 'How many times have you told our customers, "First, turn the water off at the mains"?'

He never let me forget it.

That's the trouble with being impractical in patches; it doesn't matter how sensible you are in the matters of child care, feeding the family, home economics or economies, there are certain occasions which are forever remembered in the annals of the family history whilst your normal exemplary behaviour is forgotten.

Take, for example, my driving. From the very beginning Robert regarded me as some kind of inferior being when it came to driving and in that respect was trained as a young 'male chauvinist' from a very early age. Robert himself was a natural driver and would whizz round the house on his little tricycle, missing items of furniture and my toes by fractions of inches by virtue of his impeccable steering, and performing elaborate three-point turns with a finesse unexpected in a normally rather clumsy two year old.

When I first started driving the Consul to the village for shopping, which was only at weekends, because Michael drove the car most weekdays, Michael and Robert would stand by the front door and watch me depart—or try to. For some reason, I was afraid to put my foot down as I turned round our circular drive. I always felt that I would be unable to follow the curve of the drive and shoot straight forward instead. So each little gentle tap on the accelerator would be followed by a stall and a restart of the engine. At each new start my sarcastic husband and his adoring sidekick would break into solemn applause and cries of 'Good old Mummy—Well done, Mummy!'

However, after several months of this I became quite accomplished at driving to and from the village. One day when the lane was dappled with spring sunshine, I drove back home feeling relaxed and happy. A bird hopped across my path and I allowed my eyes to follow it, feeling in tune with nature. A grating sound reminded me of the existence of a huge horse chestnut tree on the corner of our lane, whose enormous roots protruded about two feet on that corner. Considerably dampened, I took the injured beast home, and owned up to its scratched side.

'It's a good thing,' growled Michael, 'that it wasn't a new car!'

Actually, it didn't last all that much longer. It wasn't anything I did—just old age—but before long, we were buying a new old car.

This time it was an Austin A40, a much smaller car and much more manageable as far as I was concerned. Nevertheless its seat adjustment was very stiff, and it was easier to prop myself forward with our old armchair cushions which I'd also used in the Consul.

The first day I tried it out, I didn't quite realise how far I was from the pedals, and thus how little control I had over them. Accustomed to my old Consul's lethargic response to my foot, I put the A40 into first gear and one touch on the accelerator sent me shooting forward, until the left hand headlight made contact with the garage door. Luckily, the door handle was level with the light, and instead of breaking down the door, I merely broke the headlight.

'It's lucky,' said Michael with restraint when I confessed, 'that we don't spend our money on new cars.'

I've always been able to say that I've only had encounters with trees and so on, on our own private land or lane—with one exception, where I must admit I look back in sheer amazement at my own foolishness.

It was during the summer of that year, when Michael's plumbers were taking their holidays. They all had their own vehicles, which were usually in a lot better condition than anything we possessed, and preferred to park their vans in our front drive, (which they still referred to as 'the yard' rather than leave them at their homes.

Much as I disliked trying out new vehicles, it was tempting to avoid my usual walks, even though they were fewer these days, by making use of the vans.

I had to pluck up my courage to use Frank's van for the first time, warning Robert that if he moved a muscle, I wouldn't let him come with me again.

By the time Frank's holiday was over, I had built up some confidence, and was less reluctant to drive Les's van, which was the next one to be deposited outside the front door.

Michael was at home carrying out some mystery operations on the internal workings of our own car, when I took Les's van out, this time without Robert.

As I turned the bend on to the main lane, I was aware of a lack of response from the brakes at my gentle pressure. By the time I reached the T-junction on to the main road, I had to pull on the hand brake to stop the car.

I ought to have turned round—of course I ought, but the memory that flashed through my head was what had happened the last time I tried to carry out a three point turn at that point. The other ridiculous thought that occurred to me was that I ought to improvise in some way. Michael was always improvising—I remembered him driving all the way from Sonia's house without the use of the clutch, so I too would be undefeated by the car. Out on to the road I went.

There is a saying that the Lord takes care of fools and children and in this case, His ministering angels were uniformed, and driving a police car. I saw them coming towards me on the opposite side of the road, as I crept along at twenty miles an hour, with plumbing equipment—odd bits of pipe and fittings—clanking around in the back of the van.

To this day I do not know what prompted that car to turn in its tracks and follow me, but I was not more than half a mile from home when the police car overtook me and waved me down at the side of the road. I put my feet down on everything that was available, the non-existent brakes, the clutch (which apparently was the wrong thing to do) and pulled on the hand brake, and then when there were no further actions I could take, I glided forward and finally came to a halt behind the police car, with a gentle thud, as my front bumper hit their back one.

They leapt out of their car, whilst I sat paralysed, and rushed to inspect the damage, one of them crossly scolding me 'We gave you ample time to stop'.

However, they calmed down a bit when they saw that their car was unscathed.

I explained to them about the brakes, but not quite everything—I'm afraid I had to give the impression I had only just discovered that they weren't working.

'We'll have to take you home,' they said. And even then I rather foolishly asked: 'Couldn't I just turn it round and drive it straight home?'

'Oh no, madam,' they replied. 'We couldn't possibly let you do that.'

And that is how I came to appear before Michael with a very tall policeman on each side of me; and how subsequently I received my first (and only) endorsement on my driving licence; and how—to his extreme annoyance—Michael, as the owner of the van, received a similar smudge, and an even bigger fine than me.

I didn't confess the entire truth to him either, and so for some time afterwards he could be heard to say, 'I just can't understand how you could drive on to the main road without checking the brakes.'

A Crisis Passes

With increased mobility, I began to make friends locally. I developed a friendship with Carol, a girl that had once done some secretarial work for Michael and who had a son of Robert's age. Her sister Jill also had a boy, some six months older. It was a great delight to me that I could at last arrange some form of social life for Robert at the same time as enjoying pleasant adult company myself.

With the advent of spring and summer, the great outdoors beckoned, and we tended to see more of our neighbours, Doug and Beryl. On one occasion, Beryl called to me through the hedge and offered me some bean seeds, preserved from last year's crop, which apparently were an extremely good strain.

Like 'Jack', I was at a loss to know what to do with them. But I don't like things weighing on my conscience, so I dug a small hole at the side of the garden and dropped them in. To be truthful, it was more of a burial than a planting.

When I told Michael, he made me dig them up and replant them, and even then it wasn't right, and I had to dig and rake a patch of ground and put them all in again at regular intervals. Despite this lack of care, they flourished and Michael found two lengths of scrap iron and arranged a sort of metal arch for them to entwine themselves around.

The excitement of seeing these things actually green and growing brought out long buried yearnings to cultivate the soil, for I hadn't lived in a house with a garden since I was eleven years old. Now I was filled with a desire to see grass in the garden, and Michael and I went out there with various implements and started hacking away at the weeds and levelling out the bumps.

Pessimistically, Michael, (who had once suggested we concrete the entire area) decided we had better attempt to clear and seed one quarter of the garden initially and try some more another year. I thought it sounded a silly idea, but it seemed wise to dig first and argue after.

One Sunday, we could hardly bear to tear ourselves away from the task to go visiting friends, and I couldn't have been more surprised at my own attachment to the place and to the job in hand.

One day, a dark stranger knocked at our door and offered his services as a gardener. Michael seized upon him like a long lost friend, and even though I was rather sad to lose my new interest, I couldn't help but be impressed with the speed with which the garden took on a new look. Guiseppe, for such was his name, was superseded by another Guiseppe, and when once or twice a large job needed to be carried out, a whole team of brothers and cousins all apparently named Guiseppe appeared on the scene.

The soil was dug and rolled and raked and rolled again, and one day I sat on the smooth earth with Robert, peering through the hedge at Doug and Beryl's fine lawn and putting green.

'Look Robert—soon we're going to have grass like that.'

No turf for us—Guiseppe the second, with a washing up bowl under one arm, carefully broadcast the seed over the tilled soil and soon—lo and behold, the first velvety fronds of new grass appeared—a pale green haze over the entire garden. We were not to tread upon this first precious grass for many weeks, but that was a small sacrifice.

Next we bought fruit trees, which Guiseppe implanted along the edge of the newly dug vegetable garden, and rose bushes under our great trees in the centre of the drive. It was the Garden of Eden all over again.

Robert was nearly three and I hadn't done anything about play school—an essential for such an isolated child.

I received the necessary push one day, when Carol rang to say her son was starting at a newly opening play school in September and would Robert like to join him. I liked the idea of

Robert having support in the shape of friends already known to him. But there were disadvantages; the school was run in a church hall, and I wondered how much Robert would learn of Christian practices and whether he would be alienated from his Jewish background. But in the end, I found that he only learned to recite:

'Thank You for the food we eat.
Thank You for the world so sweet...'

This innocent prayer in no way conflicted with the Jewish blessings that we sometimes taught to Robert:

'Blessed art Thou, Oh Lord our God, King of the Universe, Who has created the fruit of the earth—of the vine—of the tree.

The world did indeed seem sweet that year, for so many of our problems had been solved. Michael's business was taken over, and though he sacrificed the freedom of being his own boss, it was for the security of a salaried post. We shared the car and I was no longer a prisoner in my own home, and I discovered the special joy of creation in the garden.

Everyone gave us things to grow; I was thrilled to receive dozens of daffodil bulbs from my sister-in-law, Sonia, for there is something very special to me about flowers the colour of sunshine, which show themselves when winter is only just departing.

Auntie Ethel, a keen gardener herself, gave me half a dozen rootless fuchsia cuttings from her garden in Hove, where they grew in profusion. She often took cuttings and simply stuck them in the earth and they flourished. I always regarded it as a small miracle that they would create their own roots in an attempt to survive. In fact, much of what took place in the garden was miraculous to me.

The pleasure of our efforts was marred for me by a cloud—a

small irritating worry that grew and grew as the months went by. Until I could put it out of my mind no longer.

Every time I snuggled up to Michael in the night I was conscious of a lump in his chest almost under his arm. I wasn't sure of how long it had been there—but it was too long.

Many times I had said to him, 'Shouldn't you find out about that?'

'Yes, I will—I'll get round to it some time,' came the reply.

I was in the doctor's surgery about five weeks before Christmas as I had a suspicion that I might be pregnant. Causally, I mentioned the lump.

'Should he come and see you?' I asked hesitantly.

'Yes, he must see me,' my doctor replied briskly. 'Get him to come along as soon as possible.'

In the four weeks that followed, Michael saw the doctor—attended hospital, was X-rayed, and it was arranged that he should go into hospital for exploratory surgery on the day after Boxing Day.

Unasked, the Aunts from Hove suddenly rang and offered to stay with me while Michael was in hospital, and what a lift to my spirits that was.

Michael, Robert and I spent Boxing Day with Geoffrey and Karla and most of the rest of the family. Towards the evening, it started snowing and reluctantly, we decided to leave early.

'I'm sorry to push you,' said Michael, recognising as always my enjoyment of these family 'get-togethers'. 'But we dare not take any risks about getting back tonight.'

As it happened, the roads had been efficiently cleared and we got home without difficulty. We didn't rush to get up, next morning. Even though the Aunties were coming, I thought it was more important for Michael to have an opportunity to relax rather than to have a tidy house and meal prepared.

By the end of the afternoon, the Aunties had arrived, we had eaten, and we had watched a film on the television (which by now had an aerial). Michael was almost too relaxed to be true— it was I that was on tenterhooks, for he showed no interest in getting to the hospital.

I kept warning him that he'd get told off if he was late—there were a remarkably large number of bossy hospital sisters. I warned him he must expect to stay in bed in his pyjamas and behave himself. I offered to bring him chocolates, fruit, sandwiches and, based on my father's many experiences of hospitals, eggs for breakfast.

Because of my reluctance to drive all the way back from the hospital on my own, we parked the car at Guildford Station and took a train the rest of the way. From there we walked the half mile journey to the hospital itself, in almost pitch darkness, through an area entirely covered by snow. The chest hospital, originally built for sufferers of T.B., had been placed deliberately in an area of open fields, where the air was pure. Unfortunately, as far as I was concerned, it was terrifying ly isolated.

In the warmth of the hospital, we were greeted by an attractive and pleasant young woman, who was very far from the bossy sister image that I had presented to Michael. She offered us both tea and apologetically brought Michael some poached eggs on toast, which they had tried to keep warm for him, not knowing what time he was coming in.

She went through the usual great list of questions to be answered on entering hospital, and Michael joked his way through them, so that when she got to 'Religion' and he said he was Jewish, she thought he was still joking and turned to me for verification.

Then she tried to get me a taxi, but having failed, to my surprise, she allowed Michael to take me back to the station. This was like no hospital I'd ever been in.

Unfortunately, we lost our way and arrived at a completely different station, one stop further along, and eventually parted company, waving to each other from opposite sides of the track.

When I arrived at the hospital next day, after Michael's operation, he was sleeping like a baby, but as I bustled around with my supplies of fruit and chocolate, he gradually awoke and I helped him to sit up.

The friendly sister appeared with a small glass of liquid which she proffered to Michael.

'Here's your jungle juice,' she said smiling. We were both intrigued and Michael took a tentative sip and with the facial expression of a connoisseur of wines, tasting an unusual flavour, offered it to me.

But the sister shook her head swiftly—'No, not you—not in your condition. It's just a pain killer.'

I smiled—Michael apparently hadn't been able to resist talking about the pregnancy, although it was only two months under way. Despite the hormone tablets I was now receiving from the doctor, I was wary and reluctant to tell the news to anyone until the three months hurdle had passed.

In the meantime, it was the other lump that was the subject of my concern and I now asked the sister when we would know the facts about this.

'It'll be examined by the Path. Lab. in the morning,' she told us. 'But it seems almost certain that it's just a fatty lump.'

During those few days, the Aunties ran the house, cooked meals, ironed clothes and looked after Robert, and I was able to spend hours at the hospital instead of the usual inadequate half hour.

The car behaved badly, like a dog without its master, developing a slipping clutch and a flat battery, so that each night I despaired of either starting the thing or getting it home from the station.

The Aunties, being non-drivers themselves, were not fully aware of the difficulties I was having, but they worried about me driving through the snow-covered isolated country roads, and always welcomed me home with relief at the end of each excursion. On my arrival, they had a meal waiting for me and they would tell me anecdotes of how they had coped with the household chores and how Robert had advised on where to find tea-towels and saucepans and other necessities.

Robert couldn't always quite work out which aunt was which, though Auntie Betty was short and plump and Auntie Ethel was taller and slimmer with glasses. Nevertheless, they were special to him and he was happy to act as host to them.

They in their turn, loved to tell me of the clever things he had managed to do in my absence at the hospital.

By the end of the second day, it was confirmed that the lump was benign, and when I drove home from the station, my heart was a great deal lighter.

After I had made numerous reassuring telephone calls to the family, the aunts and I played cards into the night. I got up late next morning, and before the beds had been made or Robert changed out of his pyjamas, a strange car appeared and Michael was deposited at the doorstep by a volunteer driver.

It was a wonderful surprise to have him returned to us so quickly, but I was most upset by his immediate criticism of the state of the house and Robert; he was always obsessed by un-made beds, and hated me to show up in a bad light to other people, even intimate family such as the Aunties.

Triggered off, no doubt, by a mixture of relief, irritation and pregnancy, I burst into tears, and despite the Aunties' efforts to console me, sobbed and sobbed until Michael was quite contrite.

He didn't believe that the car was unreliable, of course, and despite being warned by the hospital not to drive immediately, he took it out and arrived home some time later towed by one of the plumbers, to whom he had had to walk to get help, with that day's newspaper under his sweater to provide extra warmth in the latest snow shower.

The next day, the Aunties left, having done all they could for us. It was New Year's Eve and this time, there really did seem cause to welcome the coming year with optimism.

Rita

I had fully expected to carry on taking hormone tablets throughout my pregnancy but once my usual danger point had passed without problems, I received no more, and as the time passed my confidence expanded.

By the time I was four and a half months' pregnant, I was quite happy to contemplate a trip to Colchester with Michael to deal with a business problem. It would be a full day trip, so we decided to leave Robert with Sonia and collect him from her home in the evening.

The night before the planned trip, the telephone rang as I was watching the television. I realised from Michael's end of the conversation that it was Roger, and I remembered then that Ruth's sister Rita was in hospital having had a major operation on her hip. I had intended to write to her, but I hadn't got round to it.

I could tell from Michael's monosyllabic responses that something bad had happened. Childishly, I pretended to continue watching the television, so that I could delay the moment of knowing the truth. But I knew that only the most serious of circumstances would cause Roger to speak directly to Michael without my being called to the telephone to chat with Ruth.

Michael came off the telephone and I asked, 'What is it?'

'Carry on watching the film—I'll tell you later,' he replied.

His obvious attempts to spare my feelings and his delay in telling me the news only reinforced my intuitive knowledge that Rita, whom in our schooldays I had often called my 'adopted little sister', was dead.

Encased as she was in plaster after surgery, Rita had been unable to move. In spite of her youthful resilience, a blood clot had killed her. All the efforts of the doctors to resuscitate her had failed. And even her own tremendous spirit, which throughout her childhood had brought her through operation after operation on her polio crippled leg, had failed her this time.

It was around a year since I had last seen her, when she had unexpectedly visited us at the bungalow with a new boyfriend. My job, my marriage and her stay at University had caused us to lose contact, so that information about each other was passed through Ruth.

Now, nothing seemed to have changed and despite the knowledge that a tragedy had befallen a girl in her mid-twenties who had always had my affection and interest, I was hurt by the realisation that I could not feel the pain that was justified by the loss of a loved friend. The fact of her death was only a set of words. I could feel no difference between the death and her simple absence from my life, and because of the unreality of the situation for me, I knew I could not conceive of the pain that Ruth and her mother were experiencing.

But I had built up a store of memories over the years, and these would remain; starting with the little girl who dragged an iron-clad leg and heavy boot as she walked by the side of her tall sister to primary school; through our teenage years, when as little sisters do, she taunted and teased us, as we chatted and made cursory attempts at our homework; one well remembered occasion in 1959 when we were all teenagers, when we got off the Tube after a concert, to find ourselves stranded in one of the last of the London smogs, and had to walk the couple of miles home, dodging cars abandoned on the pavement. We insisted that she kept up with us, for with the arrogance of the young and fit, (or perhaps because instinctively we knew it was the right thing to do) we never gave her special treatment but expected the maximum effort from her. And she responded by giving it.

Sometimes in her earlier years, she was overshadowed by her clever sister, but eventually her own warm and impulsive and frequently exasperating personality had to burst through. When she had visited us, the previous year, I had seen her as a young woman at last, but now one memory came back to me—

that of a rather naughty little girl running from a family meal in a tantrum.

'We may have spoiled her,' her father had said apologetically. 'But whatever she does, she has paid for in advance!'

And now the final payment had been made with her life.

The funeral was to be the next day. They had hesitated to tell me about the death until the last moment, afraid that the news might endanger my pregnancy. We left Robert, as we had planned with Sonia. There was no doubt in my mind that we should go. If I could be of any support to Ruth then my presence was doubly necessary. But when we arrived, I saw that it was she, calm and strong, who was being the support to her mother.

I had never been to a funeral before; it was customary then for women to remain at home in Jewish burials, and most of the deaths I had been concerned with had been aunts or uncles, where there had been no reason for me to disagree with the decision of the senior women of the family.

But this time, the chief mourners, Ruth and her mother, were at the graveside declining to follow that tradition, and the other relations and friends, male and female accompanied them.

We congregated in an anteroom for the first part of the service, read out in a mixture of Hebrew and English. I looked at the haunted empty eyes of Ruth and her mother, and remembered that same look ten or more years before, when they and Rita had mourned the death of their father.

Then we went out into the bleak March day.

The coffin was laid in the ground, the Minister threw the first spadeful of earth into the grave, and the male relatives and friends prepared to follow suit as is customary, when the mother stepped forward and grasped the spade.

'May I...?' she asked and the Minister nodded assent.

She threw earth on to the coffin, saying, 'Thank you,' as if he had given her something special.

We went back to a relative's house and accepted drinks with relief after the chill of the cemetery.

Rita's many young friends, her boyfriend amongst them,

milled about amongst her few relations, already depleted by Nazi Germany. Some spoke of a small act of theirs that had given her pleasure in the last weeks. Others, no doubt, thought with guilt at the deed they had failed to do, the opportunity for ever missed, as I did about the letter I had intended to send to Rita.

I sat with her mother for a few moments as she murmured brokenly of the last painful sight of her daughter in death. I was silent. I knew no words with which to comfort her.

A Tree in Flower

In the spring of that year, as daffodils burst into life and my child gently reminded me of its existence with those first tiny movements like a butterfly trembling, my happiness could not be held back.

I felt blessed; so strongly did I feel that I had been singled out to receive this special gift of a child that I used to tell myself jokingly I had a 'Hot Line to God'.

I was busy and happy. I ordered a variety of shrubs to flower throughout the summer, in particular several rhododendrons of magnificent scarlets and purples to give the same pleasure to passers by that I had experienced on my walks to the village.

I went hunting for wallpaper too, for after two years, the emulsion was looking grubby. But before redecoration had commenced, Michael arrived home with a bombshell.

'House prices have been shooting up recently. The value of this house has probably doubled...

'Now that I'm employed by a London firm, we don't have to live here any more...

'You've often said you wanted to live nearer to a Jewish community...

'I've spoken to some estate agents. They're coming to look tomorrow.'

I couldn't help it—I just burst into tears.

Michael was amazed at my reaction. He was genuinely trying to do something which he thought would give me pleasure, though it was typical of him to act first and discuss afterwards. Nevertheless, we had talked in general terms about moving back to London many times in the days when it had not been a practical step to take. I suppose Michael had assumed my feelings had remained unchanged and that I was still an alien in the countryside. In fact, it was almost as much of a surprise to me as it was to him to discover this transformation of my feelings. I just didn't want to go. I had lived through the worst; the isolation, the cold, the darkness. Now I wanted the chance to see it at its best; it was my right. I wanted to see all the plans we had made come to fruition. The bungalow had been conceived and created by Michael and me, and like a parent, I wanted to watch its development. I wanted to pick the apples and pears and plums from the trees in my garden and see the rhododendrons flower, this year and every year. Without realising it, I had taken root here, and like one of our own mighty oaks, I could not be transplanted.

But Michael had set the wheels in motion now and despite my initial strong feelings, I agreed to allow things to take their course. There's always a glimmer of excitement about something different happening. I took to looking out of the windows expecting to see hordes of cars queueing to view the bungalow. Sometimes, I saw vehicles cruising round the circular drive, their occupants peering from windows, and I was affronted that they chose not to look inside. When prospective buyers did call, I was surprised that they did not overwhelm me with compliments, and they too were probably slightly taken aback when I told them aggressively, 'I really don't want to move at all, you know.'

We told Doug and Beryl, and they urged us to change our minds.

'When I come down that lane, I feel as if I've left the rest of the world behind,' Doug said. 'You'll never find anything else like this, you know.'

Nevertheless, we made a pilgrimage to the South London Surrey border, which seemed an appropriate area to consider, and looked. And there was nothing, just nothing that resembled our wood and its gleaming silver birches and jungle size ferns.

'Look Michael,' I complained, 'all those houses have got neighbours.'

In the period of—almost—solitary confinement, I hadn't realised how hermit-like I'd become. Now I recognised it. I loved the company of other people; I loved to have friends to visit and vice versa, but I didn't need them all the time. I was happy with my own company and the seclusion of the bungalow well suited me.

As for the problem of being in a minority group, one meeting with another Jewish mother, living four or five miles away had considerably removed many of my doubts, simply by her presence and the ability to discuss with her my apparent problems.

There didn't seem to be any reasons left why we should move, but still the house stayed on the market, and I became used to people occasionally drifting in and out, and ceased to take them seriously.

In the meantime, the pregnancy was progressing and I had to decide where to have the baby. A lot of mothers at that time had second and third confinements at home, and while, at the present time, women are often deprived of this privilege and even fight for it, it was *not* one that I sought then.

On the contrary, the thought of having Michael as both cook and nurse was quite sufficient to persuade me to seek hospitalisation for the maximum time they would have me.

When friends asked me, 'Why do you want to stay in hospital so long? *I* couldn't wait to get out,' I had to explain to them about Michael's lack of domesticity.

Being the sort of person who liked to make progress fast, he was very impatient. Given a house to build, or any similar project to organise, he was in his element, but faced with the endless trivial minutiae of running a home, he was soon irritated. In his single days, he had burned out numerous kettles, because he always wandered off to do something more interesting, before they had boiled. If left with a cooked meal to reheat in a saucepan, he would turn the gas up full, thus burning the bottom, long before the top was even warm. Even though he had lived alone for some years before I came on the scene, he never cooked for himself, preferring to go to a cafe, go to his mother (though that meant a thirty mile drive) or go without.

It was practical and totally selfish of me to choose to stay in the maternity home, where I would be provided with food, rest and clean nappies for the baby into the bargain. But with five close female relatives, Michael and Robert could do a tour of all of them and they were sure to be well fed. Consequently, I returned to the maternity home where Robert was born and to my pleasant surprise, they accepted my booking for a ten day stay.

Michael received the news of the fait accompli with a degree of puzzlement. It was becoming obvious to him that I was not seriously considering moving anywhere else during the next few months.

'Let's take the house off the market,' I said. 'We don't really want to sell it.'

I didn't feel that I was persuading Michael to do something he would come to regret, for I knew that though he was less sentimental about our home than I was, he had always loved its rural position. Especially beautiful was the path to the bungalow with its archway of trees created by the interwoven foliage overhead, which seemed to lead towards a special secret place—a clearing in the midst of the wood.

It was decided. And now I could spend the rest of the spring and summer contentedly growing fat and waiting for my baby.

The very important and much discussed 1971 Census took place and a pleasant young woman arrived to collect our form.

'Should I put three and a half people?' I asked her laughingly. I wanted the whole world to know our good news.

There were so many things to do, now that we were really sure that everything was going to be all right.

We had found the pram in a dreadful condition after nearly three years hemmed in at the back of the garage. I was sad to see it in this state, for it should never have happened. If things had gone right in the previous pregnancies, it would have been in use, instead of forgotten, behind Michael's plumbing equipment. I cleaned it up as best I could for its new occupant.

Then all the old nappies emerged and I remembered how lazy I had been about washing them when they were brand new, and how my mother-in-law had done them all while I was still in hospital after Robert's arrival. What a pleasure it was now, to see them, frayed edges and all, hanging out in the sun with all the little stretch suits and white cardigans, ready and waiting for this long awaited baby.

A couple of Jehovah's Witnesses who had visited me from time to time and argued and discussed beliefs with me, in the days when I desperately needed to talk to somebody, arrived one morning.

'I haven't time to talk to you. I'm too busy,' I told them.

'You realise the end of the world is at hand,' said one.

'In that case, I have even less time,' I said firmly, adding more gently, 'I'm expecting a baby,' as if that explained everything.

And they should have known that I felt the Lord's benevolence was focused upon me like a laser beam, and in the glow of that feeling, I was insulated from all sadness, and could no longer believe in disaster or tragedy. Perhaps all pregnant women feel that way, or perhaps it was because things seemed to be going well for the first time for some years.

But in spite of my general contentment, there were clashes of will between Robert and me. Robert was an attractive little boy, whom other adults regarded as very well behaved, but at home he was often mischievous. Perhaps he deliberately annoyed me to get my attention, because I was often in a daydream and still very slow at doing housework.

I had an old-fashioned belief in discipline, though it seemed to make no apparent impression on Robert. Once I chased him the length of the bungalow and finally cornered him in my bedroom where I proceeded to smack his bottom for what I considered a serious misdemeanour. Turning to me, apparently unhurt, he said in a stern voice, 'Mummy. Behave!'

On that occasion, I couldn't help laughing, but often I got very angry with him, because he disobeyed me. Michael would sometimes intervene when he was around, trying to cool the situation by making such comments as, 'You two are both behaving like three-year-olds.' However, such statements would only succeed in making me all the angrier. I was quite envious of Michael's relationship with Robert, for he was obviously the 'fun person', whilst I had been granted the role of 'family grumbler', and when he sided with Robert against me, it was bound to make my criticism seem unjust.

Only on rare occasions did Michael speak sternly to Robert, and one of his favourite expressions was: 'If Daddy says "No", Daddy means "No",' after which Robert would solemnly echo, 'Means no, means no'.

Michael himself used to get no little pleasure out of seeing me lose my temper, so perhaps Robert inherited this trait. Michael's own emotions were often expressed through sarcasm, and a few well chosen remarks could send me into a blazing tantrum. Adding fuel to the fire, he would say, 'You're only four inches away from me. Why are you shouting at me?'

Later he would describe the incident to friends, telling them, 'You should see Jackie, when she loses her temper; she's like a little hen, flapping her wings.'

I could always laugh at these storms afterwards, but could never convince him of the frustration of being unable to put my point of view, at the time.

Nevertheless, when I was cool, I too would describe Michael's behaviour to an amused audience and took a certain perverse pride in his eccentricities. Who else, on discovering an area of rust in the floor of our car, would have cut a hole a foot square in front of the passenger seat, with only a sheet of board to keep the passenger on the inside and the elements on the outside? Mine was the privileged position in the front passenger seat and now, being of a cautious disposition, I would sit squarely in the seat and refrain from fidgeting.

Summer had come, and it was a succession of sunny days, in which, as I grew heavier and more lethargic, I did the minimum of housework, a little pottering in the garden and, in the main, sat in a deckchair, idly chatting with friends.

But even in the most perfect of pregnancies, you become bored with the limited wardrobe, tired of carrying a lump everywhere you go, frustrated at the difficulty of reaching the far side of the kitchen worktop or cutting your own toenails. At just the right psychological moment, I had a morale booster in the shape of an evening out in London.

We had been invited to a Barmitzvah, the Jewish ceremony where a boy of thirteen is welcomed as an adult into the fold. We were not able to attend the religious ceremony itself, since we were collecting my parents from Hove so that we could take them to the evening celebration and meal.

I was able to borrow a silky trouser suit from a selection provided by Jill and Carol, and when my hair was set and face made up, I felt quite like a human being again. Most of my relations simply couldn't believe I was seven months pregnant, and they couldn't have said anything nicer than that. One cousin scolded me for smoking, but I pointed out that I didn't normally smoke many more than five a day.

After that we took my parents back to our home for a couple of days, glad to have the opportunity of showing them the progress we had made. My father, always ill at ease when away from home, put himself in an armchair with a newspaper, hoping to be left in peace.

My mother, on the other hand, regarded a stay away from home as a treat and was delighted to be shown the improvements in the decor and the new equipment in the kitchen. She went from room to room exclaiming enthusiastically about the changes.

She made a tour of the garden too and was quick to discover some dahlias I had planted earlier in the year, calling me to see them. The appearance of any new plant was a happy event, and the dahlias brought me great pleasure later in the summer, when their brilliant splashes of colour bedecked the flower beds.

Everything was so perfect that despite my happiness at being pregnant, I wished that time could stand still—it seemed incredible that in a few short weeks, this life style we had created and become accustomed to, would be changed by the new arrival. I felt a sudden resentment towards this unknown newcomer. We were happy as we were at this moment, just the two of us and Robert, whereas the first weeks of the baby's life would bring tiredness, a disorganisation of routine, numerous pressures, and a lack of time for daydreaming. There was a loving relationship between Robert and myself, despite our confrontations and I wondered if the new baby would come between us. In addition, it was difficult for me to imagine dealing with a young baby again, after nearly four years. Irrationally, I now felt we didn't need this intruder to tie us down once again and mar our relationships with each other.

But slowly, steadily and irrevocably, we progressed towards the time of its birth.

About three weeks before the expected date of arrival, Susan and Bruce arrived back in Surrey. It was nearly two years since their last visit, but the old friendship resumed just as if there had been no gap. We girls spent quite a few afternoons in the garden, talking of times past and present problems, whilst Susan's son and daughter played in the sandpit with Robert, and the latest addition struggled to join them.

Susan talked with sympathy of a woman who had lost her baby after great difficulties, and said how unfair it seemed that someone like herself could produce them so easily.

'If only I could have another baby to give to someone like that,' she said, in a dramatic statement typical of her personality.

I smiled at her extravagant generosity.

'You wouldn't be able to,' I replied, thinking of my own state and imagining myself, after all this, giving up the baby. Less than three months later, those words and the feelings of that moment would be recalled by me.

Susan's visit continued for about a fortnight and I was sure that by the end of it, the baby would have arrived. Robert, after all, had been a week early, and Susan had been so closely involved with that; I couldn't help feeling that she was almost bound to be involved with this baby too. But the day came for the family's departure, and no baby had arrived.

Determined not to have a repetition of my previous unprepared departure, my suitcase was packed more than a week before the 'E.D.A.' In addition, the baby's carry cot —a new one, for the old one's service to the four little boys of the family had finished it completely—was prepared, and placed into it was the baby's layette, carefully wrapped in a polythene bag.

Robert's suitcase was packed too, for he would be departing to whichever of his aunts or grandparents was not at present on holiday, for July/August is not the best of times for finding a foster family for a son or husband.

Even whilst congratulating myself for being so well organised on this occasion, I found that once everything was ready, I expected things to start happening immediately. When nothing happened—not during the week before and not on the correct day either, I began to feel insecure and edgy. I could only buy food for a day or so at a time and the same applied to making plans. As the days dragged on, I began irrationally to feel that the baby would never ever come out. (Very irrationally, as it happened, because my doctor was already making plans to induce the birth in a given number of days.) The feeling of inadequacy experienced at the time of my miscarriages recurred, and I felt I was a thoroughly useless example of womanhood, incapable of doing the job she was supposed to.

No longer was there any hankering to be suspended in time. Full of impatience, I couldn't wait for the first dull ache that might signal the start of labour, and I dreaded the idea that the birth might have to be started in some unnatural way.

A mere two days before the date of the proposed inducement, the dull ache arrived, but the next day it was gone. Tense and frustrated, I rang Jill.

'For goodness' sake, come over and keep me company,' I pleaded.

It was a dismal day, and I put on a plastic mac. and boots and went out into the garden and tackled the flower bed. When Jill arrived, I was angrily hacking away at the weeds with my hoe.

'If this doesn't get things moving,' I thought, 'Nothing ever will.'

Little Things

I awoke in the early hours of the following morning— the contractions were well under way and I congratulated myself on having missed the first couple of hours of labour in sleep.

I woke Michael, who was surprisingly sceptical, asking, 'Are you sure this isn't a false alarm?' although the baby was already nine days late. We sat down to a cup of tea, and left almost immediately after for the maternity home. Robert slept the sound sleep of the innocent and could be safely left for three quarters of an hour.

Outside the rain teemed down and the whole scene could well have been portrayed in a second rate film, anxious husband turning to pregnant wife—'Are the pains bad?'

Instead, my husband said to me, 'Press your feet down on the board and stop the rain blowing up through the hole in the car!'

'I'm supposed to be relaxing and breathing with the contractions,' I admonished.

Sheets of rain blew across the road.

'Shall I stop the car?' asked Michael.

'No, drive on, for goodness' sake,' I replied, impatiently. However did he imagine I was going to benefit from sitting in a stationary car? Luckily it was only a fifteen minute journey.

We were welcomed at the maternity home by a brisk midwife.

'Unpack your things and put them in that locker,' she directed me, and to Michael, 'Are you staying?' and 'Oh, what a pity,' at his negative reply.

'Couldn't you stay for a while?' I asked Michael, but he couldn't wait to make his escape and was relieved to have Robert as his excuse.

It was three thirty in the morning. How many hours, I wondered, before the baby would be born? Outside, the howls of the wind and rain were ominous.

An Asian auxiliary nurse arrived to shave me—I remembered the weeks of itching after the thirty second shave I had had at the time of Robert's birth, and requested that she treat me with gentleness. She chatted to me for about three-quarters of an hour while carrying out her duties and I was only too pleased to have company to help me pass the dragging time.

Finally, I was left alone and listened to a woman in labour in an adjacent room. Suddenly the exhortations of the midwives were followed by a baby's cry. I felt a moment of emotion, and fellow feeling with the unknown mother, followed by envy that she had reached the end of those arduous hours of labour. 'If only I was in that position.'

But a later on, I found out that there had been complications and the mother had been swiftly transported to the local hospital for treatment under anaesthetic.

The midwife hurried into my room to collect something.

'What did she have?' I asked.

'A little girl. Do you want the light turned out?'

'No. I'm not going to sleep,' I replied, remembering that other awakening in the night, when for the moment I had been aware only of pain, loneliness and darkness.

I lay on my side and tried to rub my own back, watching the clock with one eye. The pain was becoming unbearable.

'I think I want to push,' I said to the midwife and was somewhat taken aback by her reply: 'It's not awfully convenient at the moment.'

Searching through my memory for how to cope under such circumstances, I evolved a routine that included pushing my arm out into space and expelling the breath from my body to a count of, 'One, two, three, four,' and I managed to survive until the midwife reappeared, when I burst out, 'I really can't hold out much longer.'

She examined me and commented, 'You must have a high pain threshold.'

I couldn't remember what that meant, but I had a feeling it was praise and not a scolding.

'I'm going to give you an injection,' she said, 'and it will all be over in half an hour.'

I wanted to get things quite straight in my mind.

'You mean I'll be able to start pushing in half an hour?'

'You'll have the baby in half an hour!'

I glanced at the clock—just on six. At that moment a trainee midwife walked through the door. I realised she had accompanied the other mother to hospital and was now about to participate in my own delivery. Was that the reason for the delay? I was slightly incredulous.

The action of the injection was remarkable. Within minutes, I felt pleasantly drunk, and all the aching areas of my body relaxed.

It was a text book birth. In between the contractions there was no pain and I prattled away animatedly and uninhibitedly to the two women. Then, 'Here comes another one,' and I was ready to push.

When the senior midwife warned, 'Stop pushing and pant,' I knew I was nearly there. With an effort I restrained the powerful forces expelling the baby from my body. As I tried to pant, my breath came out in gasping sobs and carried on rhythmically, even as the midwife held my baby in her hands.

'Oh, that was perfect!' they exclaimed to each other. 'How different to the last birth.'

'Go on, cry,' said the younger one, still holding the baby and I heard myself sobbing still, and stopped, only then to realise that she was talking to the baby, not me at all. And for a split second, I thought, 'But what if the baby doesn't cry?'

But all was well; 'You've got a beautiful little girl; very tiny, but lovely,' they told me delightedly. 'And hardly a mark on you—just one small bruise.'

'Don't I have to have any stitches?' I asked, remembering the quarter of an hour of undignified embroidering sustained after my last labour.

'Good gracious, no!' they replied.

I was disappointed that Michael was not there to witness my triumph, for I felt I'd done a really good job, and my feeling of pride and triumph was no doubt just as silly as the feelings of inadequacy of the previous week. The pride was swiftly tempered by concern, however, when I was told the weight of my small daughter—only just over five and a half pounds— practically premature weight. Guiltily, I thought of the cigarettes I had smoked—five, or was it nearer ten a day—throughout my pregnancy. Could it have had this effect? My remorse was reinforced when the little one was placed in my arms. The bones of her arms were as thin as pencils and the skin hung from them. She was only one and a half pounds less than Robert at birth and I could not have imagined the difference that it would make.

To my great disappointment I was told that, as she was particularly small, she would spend her time in the nursery, away from the germs brought into the wards, and despite the cards flooding in, telling me what a clever girl I was, I was quite depressed during the next few days.

Although I felt fitter than after Robert's birth and, as a result of my nursery visits, was up and about much more quickly, I missed having the baby in my room. Later, when I was told to feed her three-hourly, my routine did not fit in with the other girls at all, and I used to wander off to the telephone while they were feeding their babies.

There were minor irritations too—one I'm sure shared by many new parents—the naming of the child. Not long after the birth, a young nurse had approached me to ask what the baby's name was to be. Michael and I had not made any final decisions in our prenatal discussions, so I replied cautiously, 'It might be Frances, but I haven't quite made up my mind.'

I was therefore rather peeved to find that name written on to the card attached to her cot almost immediately afterwards.

Nevertheless, I soon rang my mother to report on the probable name. I also felt that I should forewarn her of the baby's appearance.

'She's very plain, I'm afraid,' I told her, but my mother did not seem unduly concerned.

The name, however, *was* a subject of concern. In the next telephone conversation, my mother acted as spokesman.

'The family don't like "Frances",' she informed me, and though I was irritated by the family's intervention in what should have been a personal decision, I couldn't help but be influenced by this information, particularly when the lack of enthusiasm was reinforced by Michael's family.

In the bed facing me sat Elizabeth, the young woman who, following her complicated delivery on the night of my own production, had now been returned to the maternity home. She had without difficulty (and very appropriately)—named her daughter Dawn. The mother alongside me had an older daughter named Frances, which inhibited my discussion of the problem, so I spent much time silently poring over my A to Z of names.

My mother arrived to visit and I had to restrain her from telling me again (loudly) how much she didn't like 'Frances'.

'We think you should call her Elizabeth,' she informed me, and I had to explain in whispers, to avoid offending my neighbour that I really didn't like the name 'Elizabeth' all that much (it was too traditional, too 'Establishment' and in addition, it seemed rather excessively patriotic to name the baby after the Queen.

My mother, however, explained that my paternal grandmother had been Elizabeth, which reminded me that my other grandmother, who had died when I was a teenager, was named Miriam and that her name ought to be included too. I agreed to review the situation and soon a nurse brought in the young lady under discussion.

'Oh, she's beautiful,' said my mother, always a connoisseur of new babies. 'How could you say she was plain?'

I had to admit she had improved a bit since she had put on a little weight. My mother even discovered dimples in her cheeks, which I had not noticed. Robert had one dimple—two was something of a bonus.

I conducted another search through the bible of names and made my decision speedily, after a brief conversation with

Michael. I caught the Registrar on her weekly visit, thus avoiding any further family referenda on the subject, and my petite daughter was registered as Amanda—a pretty name with the meaning 'lovable' as I pointed out to everyone —Meriel—Meri after Miriam and El for Elizabeth. Then I discovered that Michael's grandfather was called Mendel which resembled Amanda, so it seemed we had effectively paid our respects to everyone that was required.

I wrote to Sonia, at present on holiday, so that she would have the news as soon as she re-entered her house. To tease her, I deliberately held back the sex of the baby until the second page of the letter, for Sonia, like everyone else in the family had hoped for a girl to join the four boy cousins.

But if I thought I could now relax and enjoy my little daughter, I was mistaken, for the latter half of my stay in the maternity home was fraught with battles with Sister, who had just returned from her holiday.

I had become aware of Sister's imminent return when the cleaners who had been remarkably restrained in the previous few days, came into the ward, caused dust to fly underneath my congratulatory cards and vacuumed and polished with uncustomary zeal and speed. In Sister's absence, everyone had apparently been having a bit of a holiday— even the expectant mothers had stopped producing, so that the mothers present had been reduced to a mere half dozen or so in number.

'You mark my words,' commented one of the midwives, 'As soon as she comes in through that door, they'll all start following her in.'

I greeted Sister politely enough, but something of a cold war soon commenced and it all started when Jill came to visit me.

Michael warned me in advance, 'She's coming prompt at three o'clock, so don't keep her waiting.' He knew that because of Amanda's three-hourly feeds, I wasn't always ready to receive visitors when the visiting hour began. Nevertheless, I rushed through the feed and after Jill had come and gone, crept into the nursery to find, not altogether unexpectedly, that Amanda was howling with hunger.

The little ward was deserted—the three girls in my room and their visitors had disappeared into the garden. I couldn't bear to think of Amanda lying there, crying hungrily until the next feed, and I took her from the cot and went back to my room and fed her again. However, just as I finished, I heard voices and within seconds was confronted by Sister. I was always in awe of her—as I had been all my life with people in positions of authority—and I couldn't behave or speak naturally to her. Instead, I behaved like a schoolgirl caught in the act of doing something naughty (and I felt very much like that), and retorted rather defiantly to her cross tone.

After that she watched me with dedicated vigilance and I often received messages to return the baby to the nursery if I took a long time over a feed. I couldn't look at it from her point of view, that a small baby wants a minimum of handling and a maximum of rest. I felt only that I was being harassed. Once I took the baby back to the nursery and reinstated her in her cot and rewrapped her in her bedclothes so fast that Sister called me back a few minutes later and showed me how to make up the bedding tidily.

The feeling of being the 'black sheep of the fourth form' persisted—in fact the ward atmosphere was very much like that of a girls' school and, despite the frustrations, frequently filled with the noise of hysterical female giggles at our own in-jokes about the staff, the food and even about my own particular position in 'the dog house'.

I dared not let Sister find out that I was intending to go to Brighton with the family (even though I felt quite sure that it was in all our best interests to get away for a few days.) My parents and aunts shared a hut on the promenade. We could sit and enjoy the fine weather, make a drink or snack lunch in the hut, and Robert would be able to enjoy the fresh air and the sea. I was due to leave the maternity home on Saturday, a convenient day for Michael to drive us all there, so I was naturally surprised and dismayed when a senior midwife approached me a couple of days beforehand, particularly as Amanda had been gaining weight steadily.

'Would you be awfully disappointed if you had to stay an extra day?' she asked. Naturally, I replied that I was prepared to do what was best for Amanda, despite my disappointment.

'Well, I should ask Sister,' she advised. 'Wait till she's had her breakfast—then she's in a good mood.'

I plucked up my courage just after Amanda had been weighed.

'Will I be able to take her home, as planned?' I queried.

Sister looked at me sharply. 'Why shouldn't you?' she snapped.

'Er, well, because of her small weight.'

'Why she's done ever so well!' exclaimed Sister. 'What more do you expect of her?'

Duly squashed, but relieved, I returned to the ward to tell the girls how, once again, I had rubbed Sister up the wrong way.

Nevertheless, I couldn't altogether quell a feeling of concern about Amanda. One day when I was sitting her up, supporting her chin with two fingers, she started to cough— I must have been practically strangling her—and I realised that I was going to have to be extra careful in my handling of her. Then there was the problem of infections—and I confided this worry to the Matron of the maternity home.

'She's been protected from germs here—but what about when she gets home? My son is always getting colds and coughs.'

For Robert had an unfortunate tendency to get tonsillitis invariably followed by bronchitis. But Matron reassured me—it seemed that their main concern was keeping Amanda away from the various germs brought in by different visitors, but there was no need to worry about the germs circulating in our own family.

On my last night I had a surprise visit, long after visiting hours, from Michael, accompanied by Robert, who looked almost grotesquely huge to me, now that I had become accustomed to Amanda's minute features. They crept in, bearing my suitcase, and luckily did not receive a chilly reception; Robert who had done a tour of all available relatives, including Mrs

Goldsmith, an 'adopted Grandma' who lived locally, clasped my hand.

'Has it really gone?' he asked.

'What?'

'Your tummy.'

'Oh yes!' I laughed. 'You feel it,' and sure enough it was—well more or less—flat.

Then the accommodating nurse on duty took him into the nursery for a peep at his little sister.

The next morning Michael arrived for the ritual departure; there was always a little farewell scene, and Sister usually carried the baby to the doorway or even the car.

As we stood making polite exchanges, Michael, never renowned for his tact, said, 'Well we'd better make a move, if we're going to Brighton today.'

I could have sunk through the floor. I knew the next line in the script before it was even uttered.

'You're not going gallivanting off to Brighton,' Sister exclaimed in horror.

I couldn't bear a repeat performance of the same argument.

'I think we'll have to reconsider that,' I said to Michael, bluffing, and hoping he would catch on quickly.

At last we made our escape. I hoped Sister wouldn't accompany us to the car, because it looked such a disgrace, but she did. However, she didn't see the hole in the floor of the car.

Then we were driving off, with me weakly giggling with relief at the scene that had taken place and wishing I could nip back and tell the girls in the ward all about it. But in the end, I never did see them again.

The first weeks with a new baby are always spent in a haze and the days in Brighton were no exception. Sometimes I sat in the seafront hut and fed Amanda, and sometimes the Aunties took Robert to the front without me, and I followed later, contentedly wheeling Amanda past gardens ornamented with enormous blue and pink hydrangeas.

Robert tricycled along the promenade, visiting neighbouring huts and occasionally playing ball with a paraplegic child in a wheelchair nearby. Frequently he persuaded the Aunties to tip-toe painfully over the shingle to paddle in the water with him, and even I, now my figure was a comfortable size, was occasionally persuaded to join him.

The holiday of sorts came to an end and we resumed our life at home, where days and nights merged together, punctuated by night time awakenings and daytime dozes, and only an occasional unusual event stood out from the monotony. Like 'Alice', I had to run very fast to stay in the same place and rarely made any progress.

I tried ringing the local primary school to find out if Robert could be admitted before his fifth birthday, but the earliest time was at the beginning of the term in which he was five and that was not for another year.

We were welcomed back in the local shops.

'And what,' one of the shopkeepers asked Robert, 'have you got that's new?'

Robert replied immediately, 'A new car.

Everyone roared with laughter; we had finally had to replace the A 40, which was beyond repair, with an old Vauxhall, and this was far more exciting and interesting to Robert than the new baby. I was relieved and glad that he was not obsessively interested in Amanda, for I hoped he would avoid the pain of extreme jealousy. When I fed her, I tried not to exclude him from the occasion, and I would invite him to make himself comfortable on my bed, as I myself did, and whilst Amanda contentedly took her feed, I would sing to him, racking my brains for inspiration and coming up with such varied concerts as songs from 'South Pacific', followed by 'My Bonny lies over the Ocean' and 'Swing Low, Sweet Chariot'.

Morning playschool and regular clinic visits somehow fitted into the scheme of things and I was happy to see that Amanda—often discontented and always hungry—was nevertheless gaining weight fast, at a rate of half a pound a week.

At weekends, the pressures abated a little. One Sunday, we displayed Amanda to our neighbours, Doug and Beryl, and they took photographs of my sleepy three-week old daughter in my arms, with Robert standing solemnly next to us, like a guard on duty.

A couple of weeks later, on our fifth wedding anniversary, I cooked a celebration dinner, and unexpectedly that night, Bruce, on a flying visit from Ireland, called in. We sat talking for hours, putting out of our minds the sinkful of washing up awaiting us and the impending two o'clock feed.

The next day, I sat in the garden, savouring the September sunshine, browsing through a garden catalogue, while Amanda was peaceful and Robert playing, visualising displays of spring bulbs in my mind's eye—something to look forward to during the winter months.

The garden played an important part in my life now. It wasn't tidy and it wasn't weeded, except when Guiseppe appeared occasionally and took it in hand, but it was a place of creation. Babies—and three year old boys too— are demanding creatures, and flowers are not. Often, I would run from the house, just to see a new bud or flower, and after a minute or two of absorbing the peace of the garden away from the call of domesticity, I would return, refreshed, only to find Robert hurriedly putting on his boots to join me. Then sometimes, to spare his disappointment, I would take him on a guided tour, pointing out the radiant dahlias flowering happily next to marguerites, a pot marigold fortuitously planted by an unknown bird, and tomatoes, at last ripening in the sun. Only the fruit trees had failed to produce their harvest.

The summer lingered on and we took another weekend trip to Brighton, but the hut was to be closed in October, and when we went there to collect a few large items for my parents in the car, the first hint of autumn was present in the grey mist from the sea.

For a very few minutes we stood chatting to one of our neighbours at the hut, before we left. She mentioned the boy in the wheelchair, who Robert had played ball with. He had been crippled by the life-saving operation he had undergone as a baby. Not for the first time, I was filled with gratitude and relief that my own baby, though tiny, was perfect.

A plague of flies filled the air, and I was glad we had put the insect net over the carry cot. We hurried away from the promenade, saying our goodbyes till next spring.

'Take care of them, Michael,' said our friend. 'You're a real family man now.'

At the First Stroke of Autumn

Autumn lived up to its reputation and, one morning, the mist was so bad that I turned the car homewards on the way to Robert's playschool, saying that I dared not go any further. Usually, the morning mists gave way to brilliantly sunny days, so that it was difficult to believe we were creeping towards winter. But even before the middle of September, Robert developed his first cold of the season. I mentioned it at my postnatal check-up.

'Is there anything I can do to stop the baby getting it?' I asked.

But the doctor shook his head, saying, 'Not a thing,' and sure enough, in less than a week, Amanda had caught it.

It couldn't have happened at a less convenient time. I was in the throes of preparing for a visit from Philippa and Colin on Sunday and a few days after that was Yom Kippur, or the Day of Atonement, the most solemn day in the Jewish calender, when even many of the least devout fast for twenty-five hours. It would be necessary to prepare special meals for the beginning and the end of the Fast, even though, on this occasion, I would merely restrict myself to eating simple foods during the day, as I was nursing a baby.

I had one dreadful night, when I was awoken constantly by Amanda crying; she was so blocked up that she was snuffling and snorting in discomfort. But in the morning, I was not sure whether to ring the doctor or not. He had not seemed to regard a cold as very serious, and I was reluctant to ask him to call unnecessarily. But I was without the car that day, and I didn't want to take the baby out in the pram to the surgery. A good middle of the road course seemed to be to ring the local Health Visitor and get her advice. She asked if the baby was taking her feed and I told her that she was; in fact it had been the only way to comfort her during the night. The Health Visitor was reassuring—there was probably little to worry about, but she would try to come to see her if she could. But the next day she telephoned apologetically; she had been too busy to call round and wondered if I still wanted her to see the baby? Amanda was so much better that I was no longer worried, and told her not to come.

I had been so concerned about the effect of the usual infections upon Amanda, that as the cold passed, I felt quite elated. Philippa and Colin's visit on the following Sunday was a great success and our two boys, Robert and David, wandered off into the woods with the two Daddies, while I fed Amanda and chatted to Philippa, herself expecting a second baby at the end of the year. Philippa, who had sent us a telegram asking, 'Can we have the wonderful recipe?' had been impressed by our cleverness at producing a daughter, and made a great fuss of Amanda, for once dressed up in a frilly pink dress instead of one of her usual flannelette nighties.

'Now that you've got a boy *and* a girl, she asked me, 'would you have another?'

'I don't know,' I answered slowly. 'I might still like to have three children, but it's too early to say yet. At the moment, I'm just glad it's all over and I don't have to have another baby tomorrow.'

When tomorrow came, I still felt a sense of relief— relief still, that Amanda was better, and relief (as always) that a day of entertaining was over and I could collapse back into my usual routine. It was raining dismally outside and it was not a day for an ambitious programme.

Michael's mother was away on holiday and that evening, we received a disturbing phone call from Sonia—things had gone hopelessly wrong, it seemed, and my mother-in-law had written unhappily from Majorca.

I was feeding the baby while they talked; she lay so contentedly in my arms, I couldn't help feeling that this was more important than anything else in the world, even family problems. Not always an easy baby, I had had occasion to say many times in the last few weeks, 'Madam Amanda, you're far from "lovable." But tonight she seemed at her best. After her feed she lay on a sheet on the floor, kicking her legs frantically, freed for the moment from the restriction of her nappy. Her eyes were alert as she followed the movements of her father. She seemed so different from the scraggy screwed-up little creature delivered less than two months ago. Her eyes were blue and her cheeks smooth and rosy and she had learned to smile all of three weeks ago.

I was quite disappointed in her, when she reverted to her normal practice of crying when I put her in the carry cot. She had been behaving so beautifully—I had quite thought she was growing out of her baby tantrums and would settle down to sleep contentedly. She'd been up quite long enough—it was nearly nine o'clock. I still had the washing up to do, and I'd left a pile of ironing on my bed, so as usual I ignored the fretful sounds and got down to work. But in the end, I was too tired to do the ironing. Michael and I just sat on the settee, and I couldn't stop chuntering on about little Amanda—how bonny, how pretty she was—how she was going to charm all the young men when she grew up—until Michael stopped me, saying, 'You'll give her a "nehora" (a curse).' I was quite surprised at him— for he didn't use all that many Jewish expressions, and wasn't normally superstitious—and I told him so. Still he was soon back to his practical self, picking up the nappy bucket and heaving the contents into the washing machine (rather than fishing them out individually as I always did). I told him it was hardly worth the bother—there were only two or three nappies in there—but he took no notice and, running true to form, was still practically ready for bed before I'd even started to undress.

The pile of unironed washing was lying on the bed. I wondered afterwards if things would have been different if I had come in earlier to collect it.

In the darkness, I wandered slowly over to the cot to check the baby. She was right up at the top of the cot, squashed into the corner.

'That doesn't look very good,' I remarked, slightly concerned.

'Ssh, you'll wake her,' said Michael.

It was only two hours since she'd gone to bed.

'She won't wake up,' I replied—then not liking the sound of the words, added, 'Not until about two o'clock, anyway.'

I bent over the cot—she was a very quiet sleeper—I couldn't hear a sound from her, and I moved her arm gently, but it fell back limply without response.

'I can't hear her breathing,' I said and put my head even closer to her. Still there was no sound.

Michael came over and I waited for him to reassure me, but after a moment he said slowly, 'There's something wrong.'

With increasing fear I turned her over on to her back. My roughness should have disturbed her, but it didn't and suddenly panic-stricken, I rushed to turn on the light. It no longer mattered if I woke her. I had to have the reassurance that all was well.

But there was no reassurance in the little face in the cot. Her eyes, closed, were dark circles sunk in the ghastly white of her face. I heard myself say, 'Oh my God!' and, as if I were an observer, thought how theatrical the words sounded.

And then quite calmly, as if an ice cold automaton had taken over from me, I went over to our bedroom telephone and dialled the doctor's number.

The impersonal tones of an operator answered.

'What number are you calling?'

I reeled off the number, including the local code.

'What exchange, caller?'

I racked my brains for a moment until the name of the exchange came to me.

'You have to give me the name, not the code,' he lectured.

For a moment the calm left me.

'Will you hurry, this is an emergency!'

He gave me the number of another doctor on call. But it seemed pointless to bring a strange doctor here from further away. Instead I dialled 999.

Michael said he would take the car to the top of the lane, so that the ambulance would know where to come. I took the baby from the carry cot and held her in my arms. Her body felt soft in the familiar flannelette nightie. Part of my mind was thinking, 'It's all a mistake; it's all going to come out all right in the end. Things like this don't happen to us. We're just normal people.'

Michael rushed back in.

'I can't get the car to start!'

'Never mind. Take the torch and walk up to the top of the lane and look out for the ambulance,' I replied, calm in the dreadful knowledge that it wasn't really going to matter.

I had never learned how to do mouth to mouth resuscitation, but I tried to breathe life into her and I gently massaged her heart. Was it my imagination? Did her skin take on a creamy colour? If she started to breathe now, would she be brain-damaged? Surely she had been without oxygen too long. But I had to try.

The ambulance arrived. The men rushed into the house and seized Amanda from me, and I, almost reluctantly, gave her up.

There were a few seconds indecision, when we realised that only one of us could go with the ambulance. Then it seemed natural that I should go and Michael should stay at home with Robert.

Automatically, I took a coat and got into the back of the ambulance. The ambulance man was trying to resuscitate the baby. All through the journey, he never stopped working on her. I was grateful for his efforts. But he must have known, as I did in my heart, that it was fruitless.

At the county hospital, I sat in a small waiting room. A very plump nurse brought me a cup of tea and I sat in front of an electric fire. The tea was sickly sweet. For a moment I thought I was going to be sick. I felt very hot, and yet incapable of removing my coat. I wished I had some cigarettes with me.

At last the nurse reappeared.

'You know what I'm going to tell you.'

'Is she...?' I couldn't say the word, the dreaded word, and I wanted her to say it, to make sure it was really true, but she didn't. She just said, 'Yes,' and added in a confidential woman-to-woman manner, 'The doctor didn't want to see you. He's very young.'

He thinks I'll be screaming and hysterical, I thought; I was only just bereaved, but already I had learned the first lesson. It was I that would make allowances for others and not vice versa.

The nurse had a long list of questions—I didn't mind answering them. It didn't feel so bad while I talked about the baby.

She talked on, telling me I could get sedatives if I needed them and tablets to stop the breast milk. I couldn't see that it mattered whether I slept or not; the baby would still be dead when I awoke.

She told me she had lost a child too—an eighteen month old baby. I looked at her with amazement. She stood in front of me, plump, matter-of-fact and motherly—proof that one could actually survive this supremely awful happening.

'How can I tell my little boy?' I asked. 'How will he take it?' I felt a single tear run down my face—the only one I had shed.

'I just told my child, "He's gone to Jesus, and we both howled.'

'What about my parents—how will I tell them?' I asked, but she just repeated what she had said.

She left me, to telephone Michael to tell him the news, and I was grateful to her for relieving me of that task.

'How will he take it?' she asked.

'He'll be all right. He's very strong.'

I sat alone in the room, in an empty void. Soon the ambulance men would come to take me home. I wished they would hurry. I wanted to be at home. The nurse had told me they were just having a cup of tea, and I did not begrudge them their break; the experience had been an ordeal for them too. Nevertheless, it seemed an age before they arrived.

'Do you want to sit in the front?' they asked.

'Yes, it was quite sickly sitting in the back,' I heard my voice reply, clearly, calmly. I got up between them and sat in the front seat, and for the twenty minutes' duration of the journey, we sat in silence, and I gazed unseeingly out into the night, as the ambulance made its way out into the country.

As we pulled into our circular drive, the house seemed ablaze with light, as Michael had once promised. Even the front garden was floodlit, and in the illuminated circle, I saw Michael in

118

jeans tinkering with the jacked-up car. It was so typical of him, I almost laughed; not for him the pacing and twiddling of thumbs. He had to be doing something.

Even the colours of the dahlias were visible and illogically, I wondered if the ambulance men had noticed them and understood that we were *normal* people—people who planted bulbs in spring and autumn—not people to whom tragedies happened.

I got out of the ambulance and fell into Michael's arms, and together we went into the house, and as I stood paralysed by numbness, Michael clumsily undid the buttons of my coat. A button fell on the floor, and I wondered when I would get round to sewing it back on—if ever.

'Oh, I'm sorry. I'm so sorry.' He said it over and over again. He was offering me sympathy, almost as if the loss was mine alone, but I understood that he could not share my grief in equal proportions. As a father, he had barely known this child of seven weeks. He could not feel a mother's pain.

It was midnight, but it was impossible to go to bed. We sat and talked until two a.m.

If only I could go back in time—there must have been something I could have changed—something I should or should not have done. Over and over again, I went over the events of the last few hours. If only I had gone into her earlier. If only I had checked her when she had been crying.

Should she have been asleep on her stomach?* Robert had always slept that way—but now I questioned my own wisdom. Yet I had only done it for her safety and comfort. I had always understood that a baby prone to sickness was more likely to choke on its own vomit if it lay on its back.*

Had she suffocated? I had read an article about babies suffocating when I was about seven months' pregnant, and had been concerned enough to ask a friend to buy a safety mattress as her gift, at the time of Amanda's birth. But in spite of this,

This is no longer regarded as correct.

when Michael told me that the police had already called and examined her bedding, I wondered what they had found. It had not even occurred to me until then that the police would have to carry out investigations, and I visualised myself at an inquest, being sharply criticised by the Coroner for negligence of some sort. Despite all my efforts, it seemed as if I had failed as a mother. Finally exhausted by torturing thoughts, I agreed to go to bed.

Outside in the darkness of the garden, three nappies were fluttering on the line, the three nappies that Michael had so efficiently deposited in the washing machine. And in the bedroom, I saw that the carry cot and the other signs of a baby had been removed, as if they had not been there a few hours before and I was moved by Michael's attempts to take away those things that might cause me more pain. But all through the rest of the night, even throughout the three or four hours of fitful sleep that I attained, the knowledge of Amanda's death and the horror in which I was suffused, never left me. With certainty, I knew I must escape from this room of memories.

'The Lord Giveth...'

We awoke early, knowing our first task would be to tell all those people who would need to know—not only our relations and friends, but the Synagogue authorities who would arrange for the burial. Later in that day would be the grim visit to the morgue.

'Go and have a bath,' said Michael, for I normally enjoyed a long soak. 'Try to relax.'

But it was impossible to loll and daydream as I normally did. Now my head was empty of dreams, and only the nightmare of yesterday filled my thoughts. Would I ever learn to forget the sight of my poor baby's dead face? The moment of discovery— the minutes leading up to it, they seemed imprinted on my brain; and the words we had uttered, like the lines of a well rehearsed play, echoing over and over again in my mind.

I dressed quickly, and soon Robert awoke and strolled into the kitchen. It was incredible to think that he had slept through the events of the night. Michael and I looked at each other. How should we begin?

'Something terrible has happened,' I told him slowly. 'The baby died in the night.'

It was the first time I had acknowledged Amanda's death aloud, and the effect of the words was like the opening of a valve. For the first time I sobbed and sobbed as I held Robert tightly, whether to comfort him or myself I was not quite sure.

But he could have no real concept of the situation—I did not expect him to grieve or mourn like an adult. The car was still not functioning, so Michael rang up Carol, whose son still attended Robert's play school, and asked if she would collect and take him. At least he would be away from the house for a couple of hours.

When her car arrived, she stood talking to Michael in the drive for a minute or two. 'She won't come in,' I thought. I wouldn't if I were her. I would have been like the doctor—too cowardly to want to face a person in that state of unmasked grief. But she did come in, and I was grateful to her for making that difficult gesture.

I remembered that she had had a relation who had lost a baby of several months old.

'How long does it last—this feeling?' I asked emotionally. 'When do you start feeling normal again?'

She thought back to the young man whose child had died. 'I think it was about six weeks before he could even speak normally,' she replied. His loss had been greater than ours, he had lost a child with a personality that he had already come to know. It would be that little bit easier for us. Nevertheless, that six weeks was a goal—a time to look forward to, when the pain might have eased just a little.

For the next two days, Carol and her sister Jill took Robert out of our house of sorrow while the grim formalities took place.

First the telephone calls to all the people who loved us most. And while I sat staring into space, Michael repeated the same words to our friends and family. But neither he nor I knew how to tell my parents, and in the end, Michael rang the Aunties to ask them to break the news. In the past I had often wished I could witness the moments when my mother and father heard of the births of their two grandchildren—my children; now I flinched at the thought of the scene when my aunts would arrive—so early in the morning—to tell of the death of one of those children.

Michael had been told by the Coroner's office to attend at the morgue that morning, and although they had not asked for me, I was reluctant to stay in the house on my own. The car still wouldn't go, so we walked down to the main road to catch the hourly bus into town. The weather was fine, (in contrast to the previous day) with just a hint of the coolness of autumn in the air, and sunshine streamed through the branches of the trees. Going on a bus together was almost like going on an outing, and to the other people on the bus, we must have looked like any other young couple, taking advantage of a day off; it seemed strange that we were not physically marked by our experience, so that strangers would turn and stare, and know that something terrible had happened to us.

When we arrived at the Coroner's office, I found that it was just as well that I had come, for Michael couldn't answer the many questions that the officer put to us courteously and gently.

'What time did you put her to bed?' 'When did she have her last feed?' 'Had she been ill?'

Although I had answered the bulk of the questions, when the officer had finished, Michael still had to sign the statement, which read: 'My wife put the baby in her carry cot...' and so on, and in spite of the other over-riding emotions, I felt a tinge of faint amusement mixed with slight irritation at this example of male chauvinism.

At the end of the interview, the officer assured us that it was a case of 'inhalation of vomit'. 'They usually are, these cases,' he informed us, mentioning in addition, that the cold she had had a few days before might also be a contributory factor. I found it difficult to believe in either possibility.

'How could she inhale vomit when she was lying face downwards?' I queried. 'Are you sure she didn't suffocate?'

He explained to us that the marks on her face indicated pressure of the bedding on her cheek, and there was no evidence to show that her nose had been restricted. But this would be confirmed by the post mortem examination, whose results would be known on the following day. And irrationally convinced as I was that I must have in some way been responsible for the death of my child, or at least have been able to prevent it, my mind would not rest easy until the verdict had been given.

But first, the formal identification. I had imagined that we would be led into another room and that we would be shown the body under a sheet, as I had seen on the television. So I was totally unprepared for the officer to stand up and, by pulling on a cord, draw back a curtain to reveal behind a glass window, Amanda, lying—almost in state—on a raised platform covered with flowing white material. In horror, I turned quickly away and sobbed against Michael.

They had done their best to make this painful moment tasteful and dignified and yet sadly I found it grotesquely macabre—this slow unveiling of the corpse—and almost wondered whether it would have been any worse to see the body in the stark reality of the morgue.

With that ordeal behind us, we stepped out into the sunshine once again, and Michael suggested we call in at the travel agent on our way through town. I didn't want to go and discuss holidays; it was the last thing I was concerned about, and in any case, I was ashamed to go in in case someone I knew might see and think we didn't care about Amanda. But it was a job that had to be done. I had already told Michael that I wanted to get away from our house, from our bedroom, where Amanda had lain in her carry cot so close to me each night. In addition, I had cold-bloodedly calculated that Michael would be less reluctant for us to start another pregnancy, if he too had had a break. For there was one overpowering thought in my mind— the straw that I clung to—I must have another baby. That was the one thing that would save me from utter despair.

And so, we went into the travel agent and with complete indifference, I agreed to join a package holiday to Majorca in a couple of weeks' time.

Later in the day, the G.P. on duty called to see us at our home. It was the same kindly Scottish woman who had called round at the time of my miscarriage. We were out in the drive when she came, searching for a nut that had fallen off the car during Michael's investigations of the previous night. It was an aimless search carried out more for the sake of doing something than of finding anything, for with Robert out and without the baby, my previously busy day was now empty.

She came into the house and we told her everything that had happened, I all the time longing for the reassurance that I had not in some way been negligent. She asked if I had been given sedatives and on hearing that I had not, mentioned that she had been sedated when her husband died, and had come out of that drugged state more wretched than before. She was not old—in her mid to late forties, perhaps. Her husband must have been a youngish man and it sounded as if his death was fairly recent. At the back of my head, I was aware that she had borne a greater tragedy than I, but at that moment, my own enveloped me completely.

I asked her if I should express the milk in my breasts, but she said it was not necessary unless I was particularly uncomfortable. I was relieved; I had found it a bitter task to try to rid myself of the milk destined for my baby; it was easier to put up with a slight discomfort. She recommended that I should cut down on drink for the time being, and I remembered that throughout the next day I would be fasting, for it was the Day of Atonement, and there was now no reason for me not to fast. That would no doubt help to dry up the milk supply.

There should have been many questions on my lips, and it is difficult to remember now whether I asked them and forgot the answers, or whether they came into my head for the first time weeks later, when the mind had begun to heal from that stunning shock.

But I did ask that one all-important question.

'Is it all right to have another baby soon?'

She was hesitant in her reply, 'You might make a replacement out of it.'

But most important to me, there was no physical reason why I should delay starting another pregnancy. And yet immediately I visualised my own terror, as I guarded the baby through its early months.

'How will I stop myself being afraid?' I asked, but she didn't know the answer any more than I did and could only reply, 'You'll manage somehow.'

Later on the Health Visitor arrived—I recalled that it was Tuesday, the day when a little troupe of mothers and babies arrived at the doctor's surgery to consult with both doctor and Health Visitor on the usual problems—I should have been amongst that number.

Of all people, I felt that the Health Visitor was the one person who might also be bearing a burden of guilt at not having called on me when I had first telephoned her. In my most logical moments, I felt that even if she had seen Amanda, the course of events would have remained unchanged. She would have given me the same assurance as on the telephone; and indeed if she had seen her two, three or even four days later, on the very day of her death, I was sure she would have pronounced Amanda fit and well. Indeed, it was difficult to believe that the cold of four days before was assumed to be a partial cause of Amanda's death. So I tried hard not to inflict any added weight of blame upon her and meted out no accusations, but merely described the events that had taken place.

'Is there anything that I can do to help?' she asked, and it came to me that there was.

'Could you go into the village shops and tell them about the baby,' I asked her, for they all knew me and I could visualise them asking, 'How's the baby?' as they always did, when I went shopping, and the unbearably painful moment of answering.

That evening, we ate a cursory meal before the start of the Fast. It was a physical effort to prepare that meal —but necessary, for we should be without food and drink for a full day.

As the minutes crept round to eleven o'clock, I became aware that it was a full twenty-four hours since our discovery of Amanda. It had been the longest day of my life.

The post mortem examination was carried out and the result was given to us on the following day.

The uniformed officer who had interviewed us, telephoned to say that the examination had shown that the death was from natural causes.

'Inhalation of vomit, coupled with acute respiratory infection,' he told Michael.

'So it was the cold,' I said, surprised, but relieved at the 'natural causes' verdict. Now at least, my fears of the further ordeal of an inquest could be put from my mind. But almost immediately it was replaced by a new guilt. Had I been negligent? Should I have taken the baby to the doctor. I was tortured by that particular thought for many months.

But in the meantime, I was aware that we had crossed a barrier; behind us the trauma of sudden, shocking, unexpected death, but now in front of us the normal trappings of death, which were not entirely unfamiliar to us; the arrangements and formalities in connection with the funeral. Michael had been told to call at the Coroner's office for the death certificate now the post mortem result was known, and when he had obtained this, the next stage of the arrangements could be commenced.

While he was out, Robert's good friends, the Goldsmiths, called to see me. The Goldsmiths were an elderly couple whom Robert had adopted as a spare local set of grandparents when Michael had put central heating in their house a year before. Some immediately recognised affinity had drawn Robert to them and vice versa, and the friendship had continued.

Now, as members of our family, albeit adopted, they came to commiserate, and Mrs Goldsmith revealed for the first time that she too had lost a baby not more than a few days old. So here was yet another person who had survived— and whose joy in life radiated from her all the time, showing no signs of a past tragedy.

It would be dishonest to pretend that I could remember in detail the events of those few days. I remember ringing Ruth to tell her the news. I remember writing to Susan in Ireland, garishly in red ballpoint, because there was no other pen handy at that moment and breaking the news in a bald statement of no more than two or three lines. I recall too ringing another friend Susan (our dentist's wife) and asking her husband to break the news to her because she was expecting her own baby soon. I remember falling asleep on the floor, curled up in a patch of warm sunlight, when Michael left me alone in the house once, and I remember going with deliberate effort to make our bed, as if it were a mammoth task like climbing a mountain.

The day of fasting passed, and I hardly noticed it, and had little inclination to eat when it was over.

Michael's mother was telephoned in Majorca, after much family discussion as to whether or not to tell her the news, and she returned home from a holiday that we already knew was giving her no pleasure.

The funeral was arranged for Friday, 1st October. Sonia rang me beforehand, weeping on the telephone.

'Oh, please don't cry, Sonia,' I begged, feeling my own tears start.

'You're crying,' she replied, accusingly.

'Yes, I know, but that's different.' Somehow, tears mixed with laughter, and we both found ourselves laughing and crying at the same time.

For the moment I was taken aback by Sonia's next request. 'Please don't go to the grounds, Jackie.' She could not know that there were no horrors for me at the burial ground. I needed no protection from this. Nothing could be worse than what had already passed.

'Oh, but I must Sonia.'

'Please don't,' she asked again.

However much I wanted to please her there was no way I could accede to her request. I, only I, had known my baby Amanda nearly a year ago, felt her growing inside me, cared for her, even then, in the womb. I had borne her and cared for her again for hours of the day of every day of her short life. And not for her sake, but for my own sake, I needed to be there with her at the end of her last journey.

'Why not Sonia?' I asked, still puzzled.

'Because I ought to be with you, and I don't want to go.'

So there was no real problem. I was relieved.

'There'll be plenty of women at the grounds, Sonia. There's no need for you to be there. Anyway, someone has got to help Philippa, and look after the children.

And this was no pretence, for Philippa, six months' pregnant herself, had willingly undertaken to receive the family back at her house after the funeral, and Robert would remain with her. Selfishly perhaps I had imposed this burden on her, but I didn't want her to suffer physically because of it.

Sonia, also relieved, was anxious to offer help in any way. A part of my brain that one might have imagined would have stopped functioning temporarily, reminded me that Robert, growing fast, had practically no clothes to wear, neither for going away, nor for the day of the funeral, when he would be seen by friends and relations.

'There is something you can do,' I said, for I had no inclination now, to go shopping for clothes. 'Buy a couple of pairs of shorts and shirts for Robert,' and Sonia, given such a task, immediately became her usual self, practical and efficient, as we discussed sizes and colours.

Our neighbours Doug and Beryl came over, and we wandered round the garden.

'You've got the photographs,' Beryl said. 'I hope they help a little.'

I nodded, not trusting myself to speak. Yes, I had these few permanent reminders of Amanda's tiny perfect features.

We examined the tomato plants whose blushing fruit we had been picking with excitement for several weeks. The leaves were faintly scorched by the first of the autumn frosts.

'We're going away,' Michael told Doug and Beryl. 'Do take anything that's any use, before the frosts ruin everything.'

'We'll keep an eye on things while you're away,' they promised.

'We don't seem to get any fruit on the trees,' we said, pausing at the plum trees. Douglas seemed to think it might be our pruning. He clipped back the two plum trees to show us how it should be done. I watched with a feeling of unreality.

Friday, the day of the funeral dawned, and it was mild and sunny. Thank goodness, for Michael possessed no dark overcoat, and I was relieved that he would not have to wear his dreadful old suedette jacket.

Driving in the sunshine to the Jewish cemetery, in the now repaired car, it felt once again as if we were going for a day out. The Indian summer of the last few days had been out of accord with my black emotions. Yet when we arrived at the cemetery, I was grateful for the bright sky and brilliant sunshine, transforming that solemn place into a pleasant garden.

On occasions in the past I had been buffeted by winds and rain at unprotected cemeteries, and at worst they had been depressing bleak places; but now I was aware of a sense of tranquillity. Always influenced by good and bad weather, I felt that this perfect autumn day had been arranged specially; it was like a sign that my daughter was welcomed and was at peace. Her grandfather was here too— Michael's father—who neither she nor I had ever met; but I was glad that he was here—if there was some meeting place, he would know her; he would care for her. The three days that had passed had been traumatic. Surely, the only thing that had protected my mind after such a shock was the unreality, the numbness, the feeling of being in contact with the outside world only through layers of cotton wool. But this day was not an ordeal. Here I was soothed by the familiar ritual, the recognisable pattern, and the sight of relations and friends of many years.

The Minister stepped forwards and asked, 'Are you the parents?'

I wondered how he knew, but I suppose we had that look — the empty eyes, revealing the mind that could not think for the pain of thinking. I had seen it myself—I had seen that look on the faces of Ruth and her mother six months ago. I had seen it on the face of an ex-neighbour whose wife was killed by a motor cyclist. And now I knew how it felt.

As we assembled in the anteroom for part of the service, I was asked if I had any particular wish. Little things become important at such a time. I asked if they could use the baby's English name, Amanda, so that despite much of the service being in Hebrew, I could recognise her name, when it was spoken.

There are no pallbearers at a Jewish funeral; the coffin is normally wheeled to the burial ground on a special trolley; but Amanda's tiny coffin was carried by the Minister in his arms.

As he strode ahead of us, my mother reached out to take my arm, but I could not share this moment with anyone but my husband. Together, hand in hand, we walked through the sunshine following the Minister bearing aloft the body of our daughter and finally stood still to witness the coffin being placed in the ground to join the other children of tragedy all around. The tears streamed unceasingly from my eyes as the men stepped forward to replace the earth. When Michael asked quietly if I wished to add a spadeful of earth, I shook my head. I remembered Ruth's mother's spontaneous gesture—the gesture of a woman who has no man to act for her. I could not compare myself to her who had lost both husband and daughter tragically and prematurely, and who had left behind who knows how many loved ones in Nazi Germany. Any imitation of that declaration of aloneness would merely be pretentious mimicry by me who stood surrounded by loving family.

The Minister's voice rang out—almost sternly: 'The Lord giveth and the Lord taketh away. Blessed be the name of the Lord.'

I did not recognise the words as the normal part of the Jewish burial service, but they were all too appropriate in our case. Amanda, much wanted, much welcomed daughter, given so recently, only to be snatched away. Amanda, ironically named after three dead great grandparents. Who could have imagined that so speedily, so prematurely, she would join them? I could see no reason in it.

Back in the anteroom, Michael and I sat, whilst one by one our relatives and friends filed past, to bend and kiss us and utter the familiar words to mourners. 'I wish you long life; I wish you long life,' and as my elderly relatives greeted me, I was filled with bitterness and a sense of incongruity that my child should die, when so many lived to a great age, and felt that the roles should have been reversed and I should have been comforting one of them.

But as the Minister and other officials stood in front of me saying, 'I wish you long life; you should have "nuchas",' (the joy that your children bring). I saw in their eyes that it was not wrong to yearn for another child, and for a moment, my heart held some hope and I wondered if I dared to dream that dream.

Philippa's mother-in-law was helping at the house; as we walked in, she covered her face with her hands.

'I can't speak,' she said emotionally, and turning away she fled to the kitchen.

Those good people; they all shared our grief in their different ways. They did not know our baby, would not remember her as a character, a personality, nor would they miss her from their lives.

But they were there in love, in affection for us. And though soon their conversation would turn to their own family news, to their businesses, their work, their financial problems, I was thankful and grateful for their presence, for the buzz of conversation that blotted out thought, and for the familiarity of known faces. I wished that I could stay in the embrace of that familiarity—not to return to Surrey, where I was still an outsider. For the moment, my much loved hideaway home held no attraction for me.

I was grateful when Philippa said she would prepare a meal for us, when the last of our friends had disappeared. She made roast beef and I realised I was famished; I had hardly eaten for four days. We ate well, and as we sat and relaxed, I tried to explain how I had been helped by the funeral. Out of horror and into grief. Grief and sorrow; they were infinitely more bearable than the nightmare that had passed, even though it would return to haunt me many times.

Eventually, we took our leave; somehow I had to learn to live in that house again, at least until next week, when we would depart for Majorca. Arrangements had been made to stay with Ruth and Roger for a day or so during the week and there would be visits to my other local friends to fill the time. More than at any other time, I needed people; I could not face the vast emptiness of bereavement on my own. Even the many letters which had been coming in were a comfort; I had not realised how desperately one yearned for comfort and sympathy from others, and I poured over the letters drawing strength from those words of warmth.

That night the telephone rang. It was Susan ringing all the way from Ireland. She had been trying to reach me all day, having received my letter; she longed to help us, asked if I would say with her in Ireland, and I explained that we were going away.

Once again, I tried to convey that the funeral had made me

feel better—better than two or three days ago. Later she was to write to me: 'Have just spoken to you on the phone—you sounded as if you had really accepted Amanda's death....'

Accepted the fact of it, yes. But for months to come, the question was repeated over and over in my mind, 'Why did it happen to me?'

Limbo

In the week that followed I learned to meet people all over again.

At the local post office, I bought a birthday card, explaining that we were going away and Robert's birthday would fall during our holiday. Impulsively, the post-mistress reached for a box of chocolate figures—popular T.V. characters.

'You give him that for his birthday.'

Her eyes were full of sympathy, but she could not put it into words.

Everyone wanted to be kind, but many could not speak easily of death. Only their eyes said, 'We're sorry, but we don't know what to say.'

It was a peculiarly English reserve. I realised this when I met a European acquaintance.

'I'm so sorry about your baby,' he said.

The tears came to my eyes and I couldn't speak, but I was glad that he had said it.

But many people studiously avoided the subject. And others felt obliged to make cheering remarks.

'Aren't you lucky,' they said, on hearing that I was going to Majorca, and they believed, I know, that they were saying the right thing. Such remarks were hurtful—even insulting—trivialising as they did the extent of my grief, implying that a mere holiday could make up for the loss of my baby. But I had to forgive them for I knew that I too had made the same dreadful mistakes—before I knew—when I was on the other side of that barrier.

How badly I had let Ruth down at our recent meetings, unrelentingly trying to be cheerful, constantly changing the subject, thus denying her the right even to speak of her sister Rita. And by that denial—not only refusing to acknowledge Rita's death and its terrible impact, but also her very existence.

Did I do it because I thought it was unhealthy to think back to a lost loved one? Did I do it to avoid the embarrassment of tears? Did I really believe that I could cheer Ruth up and with a few words drive a tragedy of such magnitude from her mind, if only for a few moments? Yes I had believed it, and now I knew how dreadfully wrong I was. Such a tragedy was not something that flitted briefly in and out of your mind. It surrounded you, engulfed you; it was there all the time, with only tiny momentary excursions into the activities of the rest of the world.

Only now did I discover the longing of the bereaved to talk about their loss, bringing the dead back to life for a moment or two through some vivid memory, briefly revisiting the days before tragedy had struck. Increasingly as the months passed, I was to recognise with shame my own past mistakes. Because talking of the tragedy itself was the greatest release of all—the greatest relief of pain, and for friends to forbid that relief, albeit through ignorance, was positively cruel.

Before the end of the week, we made our way to Ruth's new home in Hertfordshire. On our arrival, Roger greeted me by saying, 'It seems strange saying this, but you look very well.'

I knew he was right; my face was still rosy from the summer sunshine, and I still had the fullness of a nursing mother. Even after a week, milk remained in my breasts. It was as if my body had not yet learned the terrible truth.

With this family, where tragic death was no stranger, we spoke without reserve. Perhaps it was too late for me to help Ruth, but the ability to take refuge with her was certainly a support to me.

But work and life of a sort had to go on. We left their home by night, and as we sped through the darkness from north to south, we were waved to the side of the road by a police car.

'We've been caught in a speed trap,' said Michael gloomily. And I, with the feeling of one who is fated to meet with an unending stream of problems and misery recalled that Michael's driving licence already held two endorsements; one earned by my brakeless excursion into the village, and the other (about which he was equally indignant) bestowed upon him by virtue of one of his then employees driving a van with a bald tyre. Would a third endorsement for speeding mean that he would be banned from driving, I wondered?

Formalities were carried out and the policeman told Michael to bring his licence and so on to a police station the next day.

'You're going to Shrewsbury, tomorrow,' I reminded him.

'The day after, then,' requested the officer.

'We're going on holiday,' I said worriedly, wondering how he would suggest we overcome such insurmountable difficulties.

To my surprise, his manner relaxed.

'Going on holiday, eh? Where are you going? You go off and enjoy yourselves. Don't let it happen again.'

A great wave of relief spread over me; it was good to know that nice things could still happen, and I couldn't help wondering if something in our faces told him that we needed a break.

Ruth was not my only support during the few days before our holiday.

Carol and Jill, who had so unselfishly taken Robert away in those first agonising days, still had time to sit and talk, to reassure—above all to be with me; and Susan, our dentist's wife, herself expecting her first child, even she sat and talked to me, at what unknown cost to her own future piece of mind, for she must have wondered what fate had in store for her own baby, whilst I prepared for the holiday. My preparations involved washing and ironing everything that had accumulated, even the little nighties and vests that had been thrown in with the other dirty linen, many days ago. Now as I automatically ironed and folded the tiny garments, even the problem of what to do with them and all the dear little dresses seemed insoluble.

The first severe frost came to our garden before the end of the week. One morning I awoke to find the garden enveloped in mist, only faintly revealing the dark shapes of frost-singed plants. But as the mist lifted, I saw that my garden was devastated—the once brilliant dahlias and tomatoes were dramatically changed to blackened skeletons, and in its sudden transformation from high-coloured radiance to grotesque ugliness, it seemed to echo that other transformation from rosy cheeks to the pallor of death. I felt a grim satisfaction that my garden, where I had often found peace and relaxation, should now be in accord with my emotions.

Yet there, at the very depths of the pit of my bitterness, I found a small ray of hope.

I took it as a sign—as perhaps we all do, who search or long for a sign from a higher Being. In my dead garden, flat upon the ground, so that it had temporarily escaped the ravages of the frost, not more than two inches across was a young fuchsia. Its brothers and sisters had perished—it was a reminder that in nature we accept unquestioningly that the weak will die and the strong survive.

Even before Amanda had been conceived, this little plant had taken root, only to show itself now, for the first time, as if it were a reincarnation of her, or if not that, a tiny memorial here in my garden. But could it also mean that poor frail Amanda would be followed by a stronger hardier plant—one that like this fuchsia, would survive Nature's assaults.

One week after Amanda's funeral, we made preparations to depart for our holiday. The milk was cancelled and the house locked up. I had dealt with matters efficiently like an animated robot, mechanically capable of carrying out tasks it had performed before. I even left a note for the laundry man, telling him what had happened and asking him to leave Michael's dinner jacket in the porch when it had been cleaned. For it was our intention to get home in time to attend a family wedding a day or so after our return.

I had been momentarily hurt—disappointed—by my mother's reaction when I had originally said we wouldn't go to the wedding.

'It's a few weeks yet—you might feel differently then,' she had said. How could she have imagined that my feelings would have changed in such a short time. What enjoyment could I possibly get from eating, dancing and music?

Nevertheless, I realised that she was disappointed at the prospect of missing the wedding herself. She and my father relied upon Michael and me driving them to such events. It was a rare opportunity for my mother to see the family and enjoy a social occasion—a highlight in her humdrum and dreary existence—caring for my father. It would be of no consequence to me whether or not we attended. My pain would not be increased or decreased by the occasion. So I changed my mind and decided that we would go and, as previously arranged, take my parents with us, and we had planned our return from holiday with this in mind.

But now, as we set out for Majorca, the whole thing took on an air of unreality rather like the journeys out with Michael. Although I was far from happy, more numb then than hurt, it was difficult to grieve for Amanda, for she did not belong in this new setting. To a certain extent I acted out a part, managing to chat and laugh with other people in the hotel. Many of them—like us—were there to escape from some emotional upheaval. It was the end of the holiday season. Judging by the builders' rubble, the hotel was only recently completed, and it was occupied by people who had made a sudden decision in the past two or three weeks to get away; in one case, the strain of a recent bereavement, in another, a slow recovery from illness had caused them to be there—a group of refugees struggling to survive misfortune.

The hotel took on an enclosed atmosphere, like that of a hospital ward, partly because of our isolation from other local life and partly because of the gradual emptying out of the hotel at the end of the season. As a result of this, we got to know the remaining occupants more intimately each day. We were all first amused, then slightly worried to hear that our hotel would shortly be occupied by a group of 'hippies' and their leader, the Maharishi, during the second week of our stay.

Robert's birthday occurred fairly early in the holiday. We made a tentative approach to the management, but they were not eager to lay on any little treat, and though we brought out the cards from home, it was difficult to turn the day into anything special. We had a look at the hotel shop for a present, but succeeded only in finding a bucket and spade, which we had forgotten to bring from England, and a patterned peaked cap to protect him from the sun, thereafter known as his birthday hat. And thus the sad little attempt at a birthday celebration was over.

I awoke one night to the crack of thunder. High up as we were on the fourth floor, the whole building seemed to shake.

'Go and see if Robert's all right,' I whispered urgently to Michael, also awoken by the noise. For, although petrified by the sound of the storm, my sudden fear was that if Robert had not heard it, then he must, like my baby have died in his sleep.

But Michael crept back to bed saying, 'He's all right; he's fast asleep,' and I snuggled up to him and blotted out the fury of the storm and the other unspoken terrors.

The power cuts which followed accentuated the intimacy and insularity of the guests at the hotel, whilst adding nothing at all to the conveniences, not even novelty value, for power cuts were well known to us at that time. (It was under a year since we had all experienced them in England, during some industrial action, and we had fished out the gas light and other paraphernalia once again in our own home.) Now, fairly pragmatically, I added an emergency candle and box of matches to the impedimenta in my handbag. But the Majorcan power cuts had some extra annoyance to offer, apart from candlelit dinners. Without electricity, the water pumps failed to operate and we had no washing water or even water to flush the toilet. One guest was even spotted filling buckets in the ornamental fountain in the forecourt of the hotel. Michael and I were reluctant to resort to such measures as we would have had to climb the stairs to the peak of the tower block loaded with water. Obviously, the lifts stopped wherever they were during the cuts so one felt inclined to avoid them.

The longest cut of the three we experienced was a full twenty-four hours and the so-called hippies arrived one night right in the middle of this, and wearily transported their luggage up the dark staircases to their rooms.

Later, one of their number was to explain to me that if the group of people who had arrived had not studied transcendental meditation, there would have been scenes of panic when they arrived at the hotel to such a dismal reception.

I tried to imagine how a group of English people would have met this situation—for the 'hippies' were mainly young Americans—grumpily, miserably, but stoically, I told myself.

I had wondered, for a day or so, whether Fate had decreed that I should meet up with this group and whether they had something to offer me during my present crisis. But on seeing these young people wandering along clutching in their hands and regarding dreamily a single flower, or gazing sightlessly out to sea, and on hearing this particular criterion of the success of their meditation, I came to the conclusion that I could and I would cope with my problems just as well on my own.

I had skirted round the edge of my sorrow. This holiday was just a way of marking time. The full realisation of my loss would face me on my return home to my normal situation. I knew that and I was afraid. But some instinct told me I had the strength to carry me through.

The Road

The hurly burly of the flight home was followed by the rush to my parents in order to accompany them to the family wedding. I dressed carefully for the occasion showing no mark of mourning and indeed during the course of the evening I chatted and laughed (perhaps slightly hysterically) as if nothing unusual had happened to me. Did they know, those who saw me, that my body had become accustomed to acting out a part, as if it had an independent life of its own, and underneath I was still numbed by sorrow?

But the occasion was neither painful nor special, and I was satisfied that I had carried out my filial and familial duties. Now, the holiday behind me, life—normal life—stretched before me like an expanse of empty sea, with the promise of happiness, at present remote and invisible, perhaps beyond the horizon.

I was used to following established pathways with events occurring like cosy cottages along its edges, in a recognisable pattern.

Now, in order to regain that pattern, I travelled with slow steps, carrying out the most trivial of tasks from the old days, long ago, early in my pregnancy, before the cares of the house had given way to languidity, tiredness and contented laziness. Somehow I began to get back to that old routine of dusting, hoovering, sweeping and bedmaking and as I did so the lines of a hymn we used to sing at school kept coming into my head;

'The trivial round, the common task
Should furnish all we ought to ask.'

With the radio on to drown out all painful thought, 'the trivial round' was the narrow track of sanity.

Once when I was out shopping I saw the girl who had taken the census figures earlier in the year. Brightly she approached me and I realised with a kind of dread that she did not know about Amanda. Cheerfully, she asked me, 'What did you have—a boy or a girl?'

Slowly and deliberately I replied, 'I had a little girl, but she died a few weeks ago.'

Shocked, she turned away, and I equally shaken, knelt and stared at the onions and carrots in a box on the floor, desperately trying to hold back the tears and recover my composure.

Another time, I saw a local girl whose baby daughter had been born within a day or two of Amanda's birth. In other circumstances, we would have exchanged pleasantries about our two babies. As it was, I could not bear to speak to her and turned sharply away. Once I saw her baby's pram outside a shop and peeped in to test my emotions. But the baby was nothing like Amanda and I felt no impulse to seize or steal her.

The task of telling casual acquaintances who might accidently bump into me was so painful that I tried now to inform those friends who did not already know. My old boss, whom I contacted from time to time, and Michael's ex-secretary were amongst these. The latter had sent us a card, telling of the birth of her own second child—a daughter—on the very day on which Amanda was buried and I had put off contacting her.

I also wrote to the maternity home. How awful it would have been to have arrived there, pregnant again and then have to tell the news about Amanda. I had the terrible feeling that Sister would want to say, 'You fool; we entrusted you with that baby; I always knew you were incompetent,' and I waited impatiently for her reply. But when it came, it was kind, sympathetic and reassuring. Such was the weight of guilt upon me that I needed constant reassurance from every source.

But paradoxically, when people told me of other similar cases of sudden death, my feelings of guilt may have abated a little, but their place was taken by fear; fear for my future babies and even fear for those around me.

Sometimes in the night terror would overwhelm me, as it

had that night in Majorca and I would listen panic-stricken at Robert's bedside for the sound of breathing— and even as I lay next to Michael in bed, that same panic would seize me; there was no logic in it; I had lost a tiny, vulnerable baby—but at those moments, I would fear for the lives of my well built husband and perfectly normal son. I had believed we were immune to tragedy and now I felt we had lost that immunity totally.

From time to time, my mind would also turn to the feelings of concern I had had before Amanda's death.

Perhaps premonition is too strong a word, yet I had felt a foreboding, and on the passing of her cold, a premature elation as if an expected crisis had passed.

I recalled a day when whilst sorting through some linen, I had come upon some newly purchased pink sheets. My mother-in-law had seamed up my old white ones as spares for Robert's bed.

'And when these are worn out,' I had thought, 'I shall be able to use them for Amanda.' She would be out of a cot by then. Then I had stopped myself angrily for thinking so many years ahead. It seemed wrong somehow, tempting Providence.

A few weeks before that, I had had to disagree with Michael when I was sending out greetings cards for the Jewish New Year.

'I don't know why you don't get several dozen printed,' he had said, 'then you wouldn't have to worry about them every year.'

The thought had flickered through my mind that we could not know the future. A year before we had been three and now we were four, and I had had to add 'and Amanda' to the few cards printed with our names left over from last year. Who knew what changes there would be by next September.

Above all, those strangely, but perhaps accidentally significant words of the day before and the very day of Amanda's death would come into mind.

'I'm glad I don't have to have another baby tomorrow.'

'You'll give her a "nehora".'

'She won't wake up.'

Despite the many negative emotions, I went on living; life was grim; life was dismal, but time was passing.

With the return to some semblance of normal life came the sudden realisation that Amanda's death could not be put behind me and forgotten. At the time of her death I had taken no real interest in the death certificate, except that it appeared to exonerate me from blame. Now four weeks later, it became important to know about this mysterious ailment that had robbed me of my child. I recalled seeing an article in a small newspaper devoted to mothercraft and advertising baby products. The article itself was about suffocation but it was followed up by two or more indignant letters from mothers whose babies had died, not from suffocation but from Sudden Infant Death Syndrome.

These mothers each pointed out that the group of babies that died suddenly and inexplicably in the night had neither been suffocated nor asphyxiated, but had died of natural causes. A fairly short search through some old newspapers piled up in the kitchen fortunately revealed the one I required. I selected one of the mothers and wrote asking for the name of the organisation to which she belonged—The British Guild for Sudden Infant Death Study. Her reply, fairly brief, but sympathetic, came in early November, telling of her own loss, a year before, and the expected birth of another child in March of the following year. I was heartened by her decision to have another baby. She also enclosed a booklet devoted to the subject of S.I.D.S. or 'cot death' together with a form for membership of her organisation.

I was wary of the membership form, containing as it did, space for a donation—I was aware of my vulnerability, and I had no wish to fall prey to some rogue seeking to rob distraught women of large sums of money. But the booklet was so full of reassuring facts; setting out precisely the sort of emotions of guilt and fear that I was experiencing and answering the questions I would have asked, if anyone had been available to be asked. The booklet also denied firmly the possibility that S.I.D.S. victims had died from inhalation of vomit, which aspect of our own post mortem verdict had disturbed me. The good sense of the booklet won me over and albeit still hesitantly, I completed the form and enclosed a fairly small donation, so that if there was an unscrupulous rogue waiting at the other end, he would realise that there was little point in wasting his time with me.

My thirtieth birthday occurred in November, and I had never felt so old. A few short weeks ago, I had been a young woman with a new baby. Now without my baby, I felt aged.

My feelings were now reflected in my appearance too. I had no appetite, and with my suntan now faded, my face was sallow. My eyes seemed to become sore more often than usual, so that on a few occasions I had to put aside my contact lenses and wear my glasses.

Once, when Michael had accidently taken away the car keys, I walked to the village in the rain, with Robert, and as the rain dripped from my hair, and my eyes watered painfully, I did indeed look the part of the bereaved. In a shop where I was an occasional visitor, I confided in the assistant who asked me the dreaded question, 'How's your baby?'

'You have another one, dear,' she recommended when she heard. But I needed no such advice.

'Oh I will—I want to,' I replied. The gap was widening; there was no chance now of any future baby being a companion to four year old Robert. Too many years had passed, and I was bitter at the months that had been invested in pregnancy, and all for no purpose—all wasted. Except that the miscarriages had not been entirely wasted, for they had prepared me a little, and now I was able to recognise the same emotions that I had felt then. The bitterness, the bereavement, the anger, the guilt—all there as they had been before—only more so.

'To think I imagined I suffered then,' I thought wryly. 'That was just an apprenticeship.'

On the same sad autumn day, the Vicar's wife drove me and Robert home, both heavily clad in boots and coats. When I had last seen her, I had been ruddy faced, and flushed with summer heat at the end of pregnancy. I asked her if she had heard, knowing already by the expression on her face that she had.

'Yes, I was sorry to hear of your little tragedy,' she said as we settled into the car. Then she amended her words, but not before I had felt a surge of indignation at the word 'little'. It was not little to me—it was the most enormous and major event of my life—the biggest catastrophe I had had to face. I felt my loss was as great as if it had been brother, sister, parent, husband or wife. In fact, I couldn't help thinking it was greater—at least they must have lived some part of their lives, whilst Amanda had been cheated of all her life.

As we drove round the circular path, the Vicar's wife commented on the garden, all neat and tidy—all the unrestrained summer growth of perennials severely clipped back and the blackened ugly dahlias cut down. The summer was past; one must look forward to the bleak winter, with all the appearance of being under control. Once again, the garden mirrored my emotions.

Guiseppe had only just come to put the garden in order. First he had telephoned to find out where we had been, and a few days later, he had appeared one evening, not in old trousers and high waders, as we were accustomed to seeing him, but dressed in a suit, with his wife and two sons, similarly smartly dressed. They presented me with a bouquet of white flowers, with a few simple words of sympathy attached. I was touched by this gesture, so similar in a way to the behaviour of members of my own religion, who traditionally come to the house of the mourner in the week after death to comfort them. However, even we have rejected the trappings of mourning to a certain extent; and at that moment, I wished that instead of wearing jeans and sweater, I was dressed in black, in the fashion of the Italian or French peasants to show that I mourned my child.

One morning, I awoke hot and uncomfortable and found myself covered in fine spots. A wave of panic swept over me; there had been no period since Amanda's death and I had harboured a small foolish hope that I might be pregnant again; now I had visions of having German measles in early pregnancy; I must risk a deformed baby, or be forced to destroy yet another child from my womb.

I rang the doctor and to my surprise he said he would call round and see me; but when he came, he paid very little attention to the spots, (informing me briefly that it was urticaria [nettle-rash]), or indeed to the potential pregnancy. Instead he talked at length about Amanda's death, about the temptation to put a cause of death on the death certificate, even when the cause is not really obvious to the pathologist. Like the literature I had already received, he pooh-poohed the possibility of 'inhalation of vomit'. Once the child was dead, the no longer functioning body became a receptacle, and fluid was likely to move from the stomach to the lungs. He assured me that he would still recommend lying a baby on its stomach[*] to sleep, if it was comfortable that way.

I was glad of the opportunity to ask questions and be reassured about so many worrying things. The nettle-rash faded into insignificance, and yet I realised that in some way, my mind had signalled to my body that I needed help, and my body had reacted in a physical way to summon that help.

A week or so later, I received a reply from the British Guild for Sudden Infant Death Study. The Secretary, a Dr Knight, who had an impressive string of letters after his name, including something to do with pathology, had written briefly, thanking me for my donation, enclosing some more literature from his own and another larger fund-raising organisation, The Foundation for the Study of Infant Deaths, and suggesting that I mention the existence of these organisations to those who might also be in need of support. His second line ran:

'I have no other details apart from the fact that you unfortunately have suffered from the tragic "cot death" syndrome in your own family.'

I needed no second invitation to pour out details, and I described the death and all the other relevant information I

The medical profession is no longer recommending this as a general rule.

147

could think of, the times and dates of events, the weather of that period, Amanda's diet, her premature weight; Robert's cold, and so on, and within days, a reply came, full of reassurance, as long and detailed as my own.

I felt as if I had been released from a glass prison. Certainly, I had been reassured many times by those that loved me, but that was not enough; at last I was in touch with someone who understood, and who had dealt specifically with this problem many times before.

I was also struck by a couple of unlinked sentences, which seemed to be saying something that was nothing to do with Amanda's death.

Dr Knight had started his letter by saying, 'Thank you for your very detailed and clear letter...' and later, he had stated: 'We get so many letters like yours, though perhaps not so precise...' Although I was not sure that it was very important that he had bothered to mention the actual quality of the writing of my letter twice, it stayed in the back of my mind, to be remembered later.

I read his letter and attached literature over and over again, hungry for every scrap of information. The fund-raising organisation, The Foundation had so many influential and reputable names backing it that all my worries on that score were put behind me. However, I was concerned that I was perhaps taking an obsessional interest in the disease (or syndrome, as it was described) that was responsible for my daughter's death. I was a little apprehensive about showing the leaflets to my parents—I felt that their reaction would certainly be that I should put it all into the past, not dwell on it any longer. Yet my instinct told me that I could not do that. It was a wound that must be allowed to bleed freely, before being closed up. If all my emotions were bottled up inside me unexpressed, then surely they would fester. Of course, I did not think as logically as that; I merely followed my inclination, and my feelings were aired by conversation about Amanda with those good friends who would allow it, by interest in the whole problem of 'cot death' and by many tears.

But the time came for 'pulling my socks up'—putting my life in order.

The catalogue, so full of spring bulbs which I had so carefully studied, had been discarded. It was too much effort to make such a choice. Instead, still with thoughts of spring in mind, I ordered three azaleas from a local nursery. Perhaps, when they flowered in May or June, my sadness would have lessened and I would appreciate some new delight in the garden.

I had already dealt with the small amount of paperwork necessitated by Amanda's death. I had returned my family allowance book and written to the Inland Revenue. In addition, I had cashed in a one pound Premium Bond in Amanda's name, bitterly resenting the long form I had to complete for the trivial amount I was claiming. Yet I could not neglect this task. Unlikely though it was, I dreaded the possibility of receiving a prize addressed to her.

However demoralising, this tying up of loose ends, I recognise now, was part of the process of acceptance of her death.

In the spare room, which would have become Amanda's bedroom in time, was the carry cot—practically brand new—and the still serviceable baby bath, painful reminders of the might-have-beens. I longed to be rid of them, but dared not offer them to Philippa—how would she feel about putting her new baby in the carry cot where another child had died? My mother-in-law, on hearing that Philippa was preparing to buy a new carry cot, became the go-between, discovering that Philippa had no objections to the new baby, when it arrived, using the equipment, and that for my part, I was eager to be rid of it all.

When the things were finally removed, I felt a sense of relief, and indeed pleasure, that they would be used by another child of the family. When they were returned to me, they would be cleansed of the taint of tragedy.

I had too to make a decision about Amanda's pretty little dresses. So many relatives and friends had sent beautiful things for her, and I didn't know what to do with them.

I tried to remember any books that had described the death of a baby and in desperation, I thumbed through a sequel to *Anne of*

Green Gables (one of my teenage favourites) where Anne loses a baby, to see what she had done with her baby's clothes, but it only said that they put all the little garments away.

I too packed the clothes carefully away in a high cupboard. I was not after all pregnant yet, and it was too early to hope for another daughter. When I had another child, that would be time enough to decide. If I had a boy, then I would have to think of giving the dresses away, and I could not yet allow myself the luxury of dreaming that another little girl might wear them.

Once I asked Michael if he thought I ought to throw away the photographs of Amanda. He was such a practical person, I had no doubt he would give me the right answer.

'Throw them away!' he exclaimed. 'Of course not; she was part of our family, wasn't she?'

I was tremendously relieved by his reply and it reaffirmed my decision that there was no reason for us to write Amanda out of our lives as if she had never existed, no reason to try and forget her—and nothing unhealthy in thinking about her.

Nevertheless, once he said to me, 'I know it's a lot to ask, but we had a very happy home before. Will you make it so again.'

For all our sakes, then, I tried to put the torturing thoughts of that unforgettable night out of my mind for at least part of the time. And guilt too, had to be dismissed. I was fully aware of its destructive powers.

'Snap out of it,' I would tell myself, whenever I felt the familiar waves wash over me. 'No good can come out of that.'

I listened almost unceasingly to the radio—plays, gardening, news programmes, current events—and became much better-informed than I had been before, but if I listened to music, my mind wandered and the tears would soon flow; once I found myself weeping as I drove to collect Robert from playschool and had to sharply pull myself together.

Robert's life had resumed its normal pattern; we visited relations and friends, and other than having a subdued and often weepy mother, it must have seemed to him more or less like old times, before Amanda—his rival no doubt, during those first weeks of her life—was born.

Once when I was lying on my bed, he asked me to sing to him like I used to; and I tried, but I found myself singing, 'My Bonny lies over over the ocean,' and I had to stop when I came to the words 'I dreamed that my Bonny was dead'. Another time he asked me to play a very special game where we used to go out to the pram and say, 'My goodness, what have we got here?—It's a baby,' and so on, and I wondered aggressively why he couldn't understand that I didn't want to play those sorts of games any more. It was difficult not to be bad-tempered with him and I was guiltily aware of my inability to respond to his love.

On a practical level, I was rather conscious of the fact that he had missed out on his fourth birthday party— an important social occasion in his life. He had had no previous parties, but at four, I felt he was ready for one. In any case, parties are a good way of consolidating tentative friendships and Robert still needed a little help in that direction. Despite the fact that several weeks had passed since his birthday, I decided that it was not too late to hold a party, and I issued the invitations.

For the first time we had some young neighbours, living in our Colonel's old residence. One of their children—although three years older than Robert had occasionally called to play, but since Amanda's death, she had not come to us. I invited her and her brother, as well as Robert's friends from playschool, of which the two sons of Carol and Jill topped the list.

When the day came, I found myself preparing for it as if it were a major social occasion. The house was vacuumed and tidied (though everyone knows that that should be done after a party, not before), the balloons were blown up and hung up; vast quantities of food were prepared; sausages, sandwiches, jelly and cake, and parcels were hastily prepared (for 'pass the parcel'), before the first miniature V.I.P. walked through the door.

I don't know whether it was an important day for Robert but it was a very important day for me. It was more than just a tea party—it was a declaration that I was ready to rejoin the world.

Reaching Out

The dying splendour of autumn had given way to the dark evenings and bleak empty days of winter, but in spite of my efforts, sadness hung over me like a damp November mist. There are those who love the autumn and those who love the spring. I was and still am one of those who would happily exchange each bronzed or scarlet leaf for a golden daffodil, and the gloom of winter only served to accentuate my sorrow.

Now, as in past winters, I threw crumbs for the birds and as I watched the tiny bluetits pecking daintily at the morsels, I was reminded of Amanda, delicately taking her first mouthfuls from a spoon.

Philippa's second child was born in December—another boy—and I was disappointed both for her and for myself. With five boys now in the family, it seemed even more unlikely that I would bring a second girl into this masculine stronghold. Ironically, almost everyone else seemed to be producing daughters. Even the plumber, who had been my office companion in the old days, had recently fathered a daughter after having three sons.

One day he called at our house, and I forced myself through tight lips to congratulate him, as I would have done if no tragedy had occurred in my life.

As the turn of the year approached, I sent out and received Christmas cards full of cheerful greetings that I did not feel. My own religion decreed that greetings should not be sent out in the year of mourning. I could see the logic of that ruling for I felt bitter and resentful at having to express a gaiety which I did not feel, even on paper. But three months had passed. Apart from those friends in whom I had always been able to confide, to most of my acquaintances, it was long enough to have forgotten about Amanda. They had almost certainly forgotten and even if they had not, they must surely have imagined that my feelings of pain had passed. How easy it is to believe, when a person looks and behaves the same as ever, that they are over their bereavement. How should they know, who have never experienced it, of the charade it is necessary to act out and the sore heart hidden, so well hidden, underneath.

Even the knowledge that I had become pregnant again held no joy for me, only a feeling of relief that there had been no difficulty in conception. And instead of the happiness of a year ago, there was resentment that I must now face another pregnancy, and the questions still revolved around my head, 'Why, God? Why the wasted year? Why the pointless birth? What did I do to deserve such a punishment.'

Once again I sought medical help, and without delay I was given another course of hormone tablets to prevent a miscarriage. I began to feel conscious-stricken about smoking and from January onwards, I counted every single cigarette I had smoked, and noted it in my diary in an effort to smoke less. By the end of January, my average had been cut to two cigarettes a day.

I had written once again to the Guild, expressing a desire to help in some way; I knew there was nothing further they could do for me, and it seemed a natural progression to offer my help, but the thought of holding fund-raising functions was abhorrent to me. I could not expect people to attend a party or coffee morning with a mournful manner, and I was not ready for the casual chit-chat and small talk that was bound to occur.

But the Guild, it seemed, did not necessarily require such endeavours. In his reply, Dr Knight mentioned publicity—letters and articles, and immediately I knew I had been waiting for— even expecting—this suggestion. Yes, I could write. But in spite of my recognition that this was the right thing for me to do, I felt an unreasonable resentment that I, who had lost so much, must now give more.

However, the first opportunity to help came about unexpectedly. We had been staying with my parents for the weekend and I was browsing through their local paper, when I saw a short report on the sudden death of a baby. I didn't mention it in front of my parents, knowing that a familiar look of concern would cover my father's face, as if he thought I was dwelling too much on Amanda's death. However, I took that section of the paper home that night, and shyly broached the subject to Michael later.

'Do you want to telephone them?' he asked.

'Oh no, I couldn't possibly,' I replied, for I only talk to intimates with ease on the telephone, and an unsolicited call to a stranger would be an enormous embarrassment to me.

'Would you like me to do it then?' asked Michael unworriedly.

I was delighted that he was prepared to do that and Michael then ingeniously obtained the telephone number from Directory Enquiries from the little information available in the paper.

It turned out that the number he rang was that of the grandfather of the dead child, and it was to him that Michael spoke, of our own bereavement and of the help we had received from the Guild and the Foundation. The next morning we posted off the leaflets for him to show to his son and daughter-in-law, together with a brief letter from me. Within a few days, a reply arrived from both grandparents thanking us, and telling how welcome the literature had been.

It was a fairly simple letter, but I read it over and over again, warmed by it, almost elated by it. I had not realised how much I had needed that letter of thanks, indicating that the little help we had given had been appreciated. For the first time a minute grain of good had come out of our own tragedy.

Very much affected by these new emotions, I realised that each time I could help someone because of my own experience, my anger at the purposelessness of Amanda's death would diminish. I even told one of Robert's nursery school teachers about it.

'Do you intend to dedicate yourself to helping others in the same position?' she asked.

I thought about that for a moment. I was not idealistic enough to want to dedicate my life to any one thing. It sounded a bit obsessional and I hope my reply didn't sound too squashing.

'No, I intend to dedicate myself to making my family happy, but I will try to spend some time helping others as well.'

It had all begun to seem very clear now; I had no intention of becoming a crank—the road ahead led to several destinations; recreating a happy home; having another baby; but in addition, helping others in the same position and making some use of my possible talent for writing. I recognised however, that whatever I tried to do in the future, I would derive my strength from my home base, and my reply to Robert's teacher merely put that feeling into words.

Michael had acted as a signpost, never pushing me in any one direction, but guiding me when I needed help. Never once had he let slip a word of criticism about any of my dealings with Amanda, and when my doubts overcame me, as they often did, he used to say, 'I always knew you would be a good mother, and my opinion hasn't changed.'

He must have had to repeat those words many times, and I was always reassured by his complete faith in me. But in addition, I was aware of his expectation that in due course, I would stand on my own feet, and cease to lean so heavily on those around me.

My friends still rallied round me and their company and support helped me through the passing days. There came a time, however, when I recognised that I had reached a milestone, and despite my sorrow, could release my friends from the burden of succouring me; I even made an embarrassed little speech of thanks to Carol for the help she and her sister Jill had given me.

Towards the end of January 1972, Jill asked if we would like to buy her mother's car, which was due to go on the market, as her parents were introducing a new car into the family. I didn't think we could afford to become a two-car family, but Michael was all for the idea. It was sometimes very inconvenient for him to be without the car for two days a week, as he often carried heavy materials with him.

Sometimes our pre-arranged telephone signals meaning, 'I'll be home in twenty minutes,' had been misinterpreted as 'Meet me at the station,' and vice versa, and had involved us in misunderstandings and arguments.

So the purchase of the car was arranged, and in due course, I picked up a dark green Cortina, which although around six years old, was certainly the smartest and cleanest car we had possessed since we were engaged. The seat adjusted forward easily, and the steering was light after the heavy Vauxhall.

The following morning I took the car out twice, first to deliver and later to collect Robert from nursery school. On the second journey, whilst driving up the lane towards the main road, I glanced down at the petrol gauge—I had been caught out without petrol twice before, and was not going to let that happen again. As I took my eyes off the road, the car drifted over to the left, and to my horror I heard a dreadful grating sound as the side of the Cortina scraped against a short, distorted tree on the very edge of the lane. The noise was so awful, I didn't dare look, until I had arrived at school, and when I did look, the moment of truth had not been improved by the delay.

The whole of the rounded, solid nearside wing was horribly concertinaed into twisted tin. I slunk home with it and, biting my fingernails, pacing the floor, I eventually plucked up the courage to ring Michael to confess, only to find that he was out of the office.

It was impossible to stay on my own in such a state. Instead, I sought the company of my local friend, Susan, (who by now had her own petite daughter). She stayed with me, and was there when Michael arrived home to hear the news.

Michael angry was Michael at his coldest and most sarcastic. He examined the damage and turning from the awful sight, said in frigid tones, 'It's up to you, if you want to spoil your little toys.'

For the next few days, until a repair was carried out and the physical reminders of my misdemeanour removed, he could only speak of the incident with such chilly and biting comments.

I was surprised that after all we had been through, we could both still get so upset about an inanimate object like a car. I felt almost relieved that we could. Nevertheless, I got very attached to the Cortina after that and was grateful for its permanent availability. Thereafter, I was eminently careful with it for some time.

It was not until the end of February that I began to take my pregnancy seriously. Of course, I had taken my hormone tablets and other necessary pills as a matter of course, and I had managed to maintain my average of two cigarettes a day. But I didn't feel pregnant, for in fact, in all my five pregnancies I was one of those lucky people who experiences no nausea or other unpleasant side effects during the first three months. Since there was no 'bump' nor any movement at that stage, it was easy to forget I was pregnant until the fourth month.

At the crucial three-month point, however, I did one day get rather panicky and upset.

Michael was unsympathetic, and asked aggressively, 'Are you going to go on like this for the whole of this pregnancy?'

I was indignant at his lack of understanding, particularly as I felt I had done rather well, all things considered. Nevertheless, mustering my dignity and trying to control my sobs, for he really couldn't bear me to be in an emotional state and was quite likely to walk out until I'd calmed down, I tried to express my feelings in the sort of practical terms he would understand.

'Imagine you were building a house,' I said, remembering the time when we were constructing the bungalow, 'and you got to window height, and vandals came along and knocked it down; then the same thing happened a second time; finally, you succeeded in completing the whole house, right up to the top, and it was destroyed again, how would you feel, when you came to trying it again?'

I think he understood, but in fact I think he'd really understood all along; he just didn't want to see me in a permanently tense state about the pregnancy. But his concern was unnecessary, for once I had passed the three-month hurdle, I was able to become more relaxed. I had not experienced problems in the latter part of pregnancy and there was no cause for me to think I would start now. No, there was no reason to feel uneasy until the baby was in my arms; and then I would face a new set of worries.

The baby was due at the end of August and we might have expected to hold the consecration of Amanda's tombstone (an occasion which tends to represent the end of the mourning period) not long after that—a year after her death. But with a new baby making its own demands on me, how would I give Amanda my full attention? I decided instead that we should have the ceremony when I was seven months' pregnant; any later than that, I should be reluctant to travel from Surrey to Hertfordshire where Amanda was buried. So although it was now only March, I went to London to select the tombstone and the wording and arrange the date of the consecration in June.

I also made a trip to the maternity home to book up my stay there. As I had anticipated there were no difficulties in doing this, although there were some painful moments as a young nurse took notes of my gynaecological history:

1967—Son born
1969—Miscarriage
1970—Miscarriage
1971—Daughter born—died at seven weeks

When she reached the end of this section of the notes, she breathed a sigh of relief, as if to say, 'That's got rid of that unpleasant part.'

I thought she might have made some small sympathetic comment. I was quite surprised that a nurse trained to deal so specifically with the bringing about of life, could not also have some knowledge of how to deal with misfortune or death.

I had not forgotten my decision to try to write about the subject of 'cot death'. Things might be different after this baby was born, so I had to begin without delay. It seemed logical, initially, to get something into the local church Newsletter, for here in the village, I was immediately available to anyone in the same distress that I had experienced. Then I hoped to put something in our synagogue Newsletter, which was always interested in contributions. After that I could attempt the much harder task of letters to the press and newspaper or magazine articles and ultimately, perhaps even a book.

Cautiously I started at the bottom rung of my own stepladder, by composing a letter to the people of the village, and the tapping of the typewriter in the spare room became a common sound as I amended my work. Since the parish Newsletter was a single sheet of paper folded to form four sides of writing, it was perhaps a little optimistic of me to hope that the vicar would include it.

So I was pleased and surprised to receive a visit from him, not long after I had forwarded my letter to him.

He was a very tall man, and had to duck to avoid hitting his head on the chandelier, and I sat uncomfortably aware of his height and the dignity of his position in the church, as we discussed the possibility of printing the letter in the next two or three months. It is difficult to know whether I would have been more or less embarrassed had he been a rabbi instead.

I began working then on an article for the synagogue Newsletter. The tears would flow as I sat at the typewriter recalling that sad time and it took weeks of typing and retyping to achieve the finished product I desired. But the tears were not destructive. I would reach a point where I was emotionally drained and I would wipe my eyes and walk from the room. And yet at the same time, I felt satisfied, and I was able to recover my composure quite quickly.

By the time I was four months pregnant, I was smoking less than two cigarettes a day, sometimes none at all. I have heard of revulsion therapy—and in my own case, I became increasingly disgusted by the habit until finally even the taste of a cigarette became unpleasant to me. I did not invite this feeling, and even though at the time, it was not suggested that smoking was directly implicated in cot death,[*] I could not put out of my mind

*Note: *Current guidelines recommend that to help lower the risk of cot death, smoking is totally avoided both during and after pregnancy.*

159

the accusing voice that said, 'How can you bear to endanger *this* baby in any way?' And so finally at the beginning of April, I smoked my last cigarette.

As Easter and the Jewish Passover approached, I made up my mind to hold the family Passover meal and service in my home for the first time.

A table was prepared, upon which certain foods were placed—the unleavened bread, salt water for tears, the lamb bone representing the sacrificial offering, the bitter herb to remind us of the hardship undergone by our forefathers, the egg symbolising the continuity of life itself. During the service, the father would point to each item and explain its significance to the children.

And when the story was told, there was the family dinner, a meal traditionally to be enjoyed in the knowledge that we were free men and women.

There was quite a lot of work to do, and the family may well have wondered why I chose that particular year to do it. To a certain extent, the reason for my decision to take this on was similar to that which pushed me into holding Robert's belated birthday party—a desire to show everyone that life was going on in our house. But additionally, I wanted to demonstrate that I had not become so embittered as to wish to forget the traditions of my religion. Indeed as I sought to create something good out of Amanda's death, I became less bitter, and even began to think that far from being punished, I had been chosen to carry out the task of helping other young women like myself, either through direct contact with them or through writing about cot death and bringing the support groups to their notice.

However, it was not until May that the first of my efforts bore fruit, and my letter, slightly edited by the Vicar, in order to fit into the slim parish Newsletter, was printed.

Within a day or so another letter of mine, written quite spontaneously following a programme on cot death, was broadcast on the radio. Cot death was beginning to be a better publicised subject by then and yet the Foundation and the Guild had only been conceived in 1970. Before that time, the mothers of a thousand or more dead babies a year had been quite alone, not only unsupported, but often accused of negligence or worse. I thanked heaven that Amanda, if she had to die, had died in 1971.

And now, almost nine months later on the 25th June, 1972, the memorial stone to Amanda was consecrated in a traditional Jewish ceremony. Shaken with tears, I said my last 'Goodbye' to her. 'Goodbye', for when I next visited the tombstone, it was just a quiet empty place with no presence there any longer; and I shed no tears. But by that time I had written Amanda's name in many letters and spoken it in many places and the inscribed piece of stone was not her only memorial.

After the ceremony, once again Philippa and Colin received us all at their home. Once again, I had asked a great deal of them, but they had willingly opened their house and provided refreshments for many of our friends and relations. Later, when all but our own family had gone, we ate a hearty meal, and the day developed into a normal family occasion. The little boys, with the exception of six month old baby Mark played happily while the adults gossiped. At the end of the day when we left, Michael's brother Geoffrey said to Philippa: 'It's been a lovely day,' and for the moment, I was hurt, for it seemed they had all forgotten how the day had started. But he was right. It had been a happy day, after all. The family had radiated its usual warmth, and I could not help but be relaxed and happy amongst them. Spring had come and the ice around my heart had melted.

Delivery

It is difficult to say quite when the change had taken place in me. The daffodils had bloomed, but my heart had remained heavy; then the red dogwood had been dotted with new shoots, the dry, deciduous sticks of hawthorn became fringed with green, the apple trees and the plum trees had borne blossom, and the garden had burst into life. Even the tiny fuchsia, lost in the frosts of winter, had reappeared. And suddenly I knew that I had come through a long dark tunnel and I had survived. Even though my child was yet unborn, and there were a new set of fears ahead of me, I knew my ordeal of pain was past. I had thought I would be bitter and scarred for life, and I had been wrong. I had thought I would never laugh again, and I was wrong. I had not been destroyed, I had been strengthened; my life had not been ruined, it had been rerouted.

But even this awareness could not prevent the fairly normal feelings of irritation at the moderate discomfort I experienced. Now in August, I waddled around feeling plump, heavy and resentful near the end of another summer pregnancy. I was plagued with heartburn, an affliction particularly reserved for short, pregnant women, I feel sure, and tired after what seemed like an eternity, and what was after all, nearly two years of pregnancy with only a short break in the middle.

It was a year since that summer when I had been so full of happiness awaiting the birth of my child, yet fearful of the effect of her arrival on our relationships with each other. I looked back to my ecstatic pleasure in carrying out the preparations for the baby's arrival with some cynicism, and had little energy or enthusiasm to prepare the layette and nappies this time.

This pregnancy, almost completely joyless, was purely a necessary evil. I waited now, as for the missing piece of a jigsaw to complete the picture.

Amanda had been a small visitor who had totally disorganised the pleasant pattern of our lives, yet her death had caused a great gaping chasm, and, without her, our family had become suddenly incomplete.

I tried to stem the longing for a daughter to replace her and prayed first for a fit and healthy child, and only after that—if possible—a little girl. My awareness of all the potential dangers was heightened, and I was afraid to hope for too much.

I still felt a kind of fear at the new ties that threatened the spontaneity of our lives, but this time, Robert's impending exodus to school would impose much greater restrictions than the arrival of the new baby.

Visits to the doctor for preschool jabs were fitted in with all the usual prenatal check-ups.

'Is this going to be another small baby?' I asked the doctor, worriedly on one of the later visits.

'It could be,' he admitted. 'I should hold on to it as long as possible.' Robert had made a formal visit to school, and he was so overwhelmed by the large amount of children, that he had hidden behind me, clinging to my skirt.

I told the headmaster that Robert's baby sister already recorded in his notes had died.

'I know,' he said. 'I read your letter in the Newsletter.'

He gave me the details of the school terms, showing that Robert would be required to start school on 6th September; the new baby was due on 25th August, but could so easily be a week or more late. I asked whether, if I was still in hospital, Robert could miss the first few days of school. The headmaster was dubious at the time, but later he rang me to tell me that Robert's class were being put in a newly built classroom, which would not be ready until September 11th. To avoid confusing the little ones, he had decided it would be better for them to start on the 11th and not the 6th September. This was a bonus, and I didn't know whether to thank the Fates who had organised it, or the headmaster, for finding a way out of my own difficulty.

The very weekend before the baby was due, we were invited to a party by Jill, who was moving house. I couldn't even remember the last time I had been to a party, and our neighbours, Doug and Beryl offered to babysit, as their teenage daughter was already booked. My tiredness evaporated and I stood happily talking, sipping drinks without my customary heartburn. A figure from my past walked in—a young man from my happy days at a Mayfair office, more than six years ago. I asked after his wife.

'We broke up,' he told me. 'We're divorced.'

'I'm sorry,' I said, remembering what an attractive couple they had made. 'Were there any children?'

'No,' he replied, saying then, 'I suppose there are lots of little Lubens at home.'

I told him then about Robert and the miscarriages and poor little Amanda.

'You've been very unlucky,' he commented sympathetically.

I thought about the empty, broken shell of his marriage, which had looked as if it had all the ingredients for success. I compared it with our own marriage, woven with strands of disappointment and triumph, and enriched by the sharing of pain and happiness, blessed by our son Robert and the new child waiting to be born so soon now, and quite spontaneously I said, 'No, we've been very lucky.'

I lay in bed; I was damp and sweaty, my back aching.

'I think the waters have broken,' I said, getting out of bed, but they hadn't.

It was five o'clock in the morning; I woke up.

'The waters have broken,' I told Michael.

'Are you sure this isn't a false alarm?' he said crossly, unable to get back to sleep, once he was disturbed.

'No, I'm quite sure,' I said, but I didn't know what to do. It was two days early and the doctor had said, 'Hold on to it for as long as possible'. If I went into hospital now, they would give me an enema, and things would start moving.

Foolishly I dithered, wondering whether to phone them or not.

Michael, always impatient with indecisiveness, got up, showered and dressed himself.

'What are you going to do?' I enquired.

'I'm going to repair the car,' he replied. 'I can't stand around doing nothing.'

I didn't try too hard to dissuade him and he disappeared outside the door to adjust the brakes on the old Vauxhall—they had been becoming a little slack in the past few days.

He was no asset to have around on such occasions; he was too impatient ever to be a calming influence; it was really much easier to let him go off and busy himself with some useful job than to put up with being hurried and chivied along.

Left now to my own devices, I decided to telephone the maternity home; the night staff were shortly coming off duty and since there was no urgency, I was told to come in at my leisure.

As I lay back on my bed, I heard a dull thud outside, and I assumed it was Michael tinkering with his car. I couldn't be bothered to get up and look out of the window to see what he was doing, but some minutes later he appeared and practically flung himself on the bed, his face contorted with pain.

'Whatever is it?' I asked in alarm.

'The car fell on my foot—the jack slipped,' he explained.

I didn't know how to help him; he was obviously in so much greater pain than I was going to be in the course of the day. All I could do was hold him to me and try to comfort him. I could have wept for him. At the same time, I couldn't help being slightly irritated; this, after all, was my day for the attention and fussing; I wanted a useful and reliable husband around, not someone getting into scrapes and needing help himself.

Nevertheless, he did recover some of his equilibrium soon, and began to make himself some breakfast (I had no stomach for it,) congratulating me on the way the food and utensils were positioned, for he was able to carry out the entire egg-boiling and eating operation from almost one spot in the kitchen.

In the meantime, I had received a telephone call.

'What's this I hear, Mrs Luben?' came the familiar tones of Sister. 'You've had one contraction and you want to come in?'

'I didn't say that at all,' I replied indignantly. 'I haven't had any contractions, but the waters have broken.' I knew as well as she did that the baby had now lost its sterile protection, and that that was the reason for going into hospital, not necessarily because the birth (or even labour) was imminent.

With the misunderstanding cleared up, she said I could come in, but I explained about Michael's injured foot, and managing to sound rather efficient, asked if I could first get the household organised before my departure.

I didn't actually do very much except make one or two telephone calls. I couldn't resist telephoning the doctor, to make sure it was really all right for me to go into the maternity home and start the chain of events leading up to labour. He must have thought I was being rather foolish to ask; for who can stop Nature in her tracks at that stage?

Luckily, he was able to make an appointment to see Michael's foot at the time when I should myself have been visiting him for a normal check-up.

Robert got up from bed, and received stern warning to stay away from both of us. At nearly five years old, he was one of those boys who almost always walk into or over things rather than around them; neither of us felt like being bumped into, and he would certainly have trodden on Michael's injured foot if allowed within three yards of it.

Now we had to decide which of the relations to dispatch him to—Michael was hardly in a fit state to drive very far, but luckily the Cortina only needed one foot to operate it.

Our first approach was made to our good friends, the Goldsmiths, and our disappointment was great on hearing they were going to London. However, inspiration dawned, and we asked them to deposit Robert at Philippa's house in London, thereafter to be transferred to any other available bit of family.

Before long, I arrived at the maternity home, complete with suitcase and injured husband, with a feeling of relief that now matters would be taken out of my hands and things would soon be under way. I had seen cases where women had spent two days in hospital after the waters had broken, waiting unhappily for labour to commence, but I had already felt the first faint contractions and hoped that I would not fall into that category.

Twice I had borne the pangs of labour in the lonely darkness of the night, and only after the first light of the morning had my children been born. Now outside the window, almost remote from me, the sun was shining in a clear blue sky; it was a fine August day, one of the few, it seemed to me, in that fairly dull summer; it boded well for my child.

Labour carried out to the accompaniment of lunch, tea and the busy atmosphere of the day was a much more prosaic affair than those two solitary nights I had experienced.

Michael hobbled back, not long after his visit to the doctor. Mercifully, his foot, now vastly swollen and clad only in a sock (his shoe was still under the car) was merely bruised and no bones appeared to be broken.

'Where's Mrs Luben?' I heard Sister's voice ring out. 'She can take her husband for a walk around the garden—oh, no. He can't walk.'

I was glad to be let off the hook as I had no wish to spend the day walking round the garden with or without Michael, particularly if it involved meeting up with women who had already given birth some days ago.

The contractions were not too bad at that stage; I observed them with an almost clinical interest. It was as if a giant hand had caught hold of a part of me, located somewhere in the centre of my anatomy and was gently squeezing it.

It was sensible to begin breathing correctly now, before the contractions became more acute.

Michael didn't stay long after that; at the first signs of me breathing through a contraction, he said, 'What are you making all those funny faces for?'

He'd been through all the breathing exercises with me,

during the first pregnancy, but he still behaved as if I was putting on an act! Spending the day with me in labour was definitely not his favourite occupation, and before long he had deserted me.

I was in an intimate two-bed ward, the same room and bed, in fact, where I had spent ten days after Robert's birth. My roommate was marginally ahead of me; we sat champing through our lunches watching each other's faces for signs of contractions.

Her husband, who wanted to be present at the birth, was located mid-afternoon, by which time her pains were getting stronger. Screened from my view, I nevertheless heard her discomfort increase, until Sister popped in with official visitors; she glanced just once at my neighbour, and immediately called: 'Nurse! Get Mrs Taylor to the delivery room.'

I was impressed by the speed of her diagnosis, and heard later that she was a remarkably kind midwife too; it had not occurred to me before that she ever officiated at a delivery.

My neighbour's husband, en passant, asked me how I was feeling.

'I think I'm a couple of hours behind your wife,' I answered weakly. The giant hand was squeezing ruthlessly now, sadistically.

I had spent much of the afternoon sitting in a chair, carefully timing the contractions; by this time I was lying in bed, no longer able to sit up comfortably.

To break the monotony, I walked to the loo, at half past each hour, and on the hour, a pleasant Indian nurse visited me.

'You must have your baby by seven o'clock,' she told me, 'and then you will have a girl; the last baby I delivered was a boy and so the next will be a girl. But I go off duty at seven.'

'I'll try and have it by seven o'clock,' I promised, hoping sincerely that labour would not be extended beyond that time, in view of my increasing discomfort. But apart from that, I had no wish to lose the support of this nurse who had been observing me all day. In addition, even though I knew the baby's sex had been determined nine months ago, we all get a little super-stitious sometimes.

At five-thirty, I dragged myself weakly to the toilet once again, but by six o'clock, I was praying for the arrival of my nurse; I should have rung for her; now I had left things so late, that I could hardly walk, and had to be helped to the delivery room.

Every part of my body was throbbing, and I had no control over it except the bit that was pushing the baby out. My hand gripped the wrist of the staff nurse in charge, and to my embarrassment I couldn't release it.

'She's having a spasm,' said the staff nurse, prising my fingers away. 'Do you want gas and air?'

I wanted to answer her politely, 'Yes please, if you think it will help,' but no sound came out of my mouth. I knew I was doing something wrong—over-breathing, under-breathing or something; I had failed to re-read my 'natural childbirth' book—I had had no heart for it, and as a result, this would not be the perfect birth as Amanda's had been. I was completely overpowered by the contractions and the vibrations of every nerve-end of my body. I felt like a musical instrument that was being harshly played; geometric patterns concertinaing open and closed in time with the vibrations flashed through my mind.

Then suddenly, miraculously, we were there, with that unforgettable sensation of the baby sliding into the world.

The vibrations stopped; my body returned into my possession.

It was several seconds before I could appreciate the miracle that had happened. I had given birth to a daughter.

'Thank goodness I don't have to do that again,' I murmured.

The Indian nurse looked surprised. 'But there were only three contractions,' she pointed out.

'Oh but what contractions!' was all I could reply.

I soon recovered enough to ask the baby's weight. Relief flooded over me when I heard she weighed six pound five ounces. This was not an abnormally small weight; it was only seven

ounces less than Robert at birth—and I was a small woman—
not meant to produce large babies.

When the little one was placed in my arms, I saw at once that
her arms and legs were plump and shapely, and the tiny fingers
and elbows dimpled like those of a doll. And now that I was a
better judge of the screwed up faces of new born babies, I could
see that she was quite a beauty.

Before I had left the delivery room, Michael strolled in un-
hurriedly. I saw at once that he had no idea the baby had arrived. I tried to bluff it out for a few moments, but I couldn't
keep it up. I had no strength for games at the moment. I was
nauseous and drained and faintly irritated with myself for al-
lowing errors in judgement to spoil the last moments of birth. I
felt regretful, too, that Michael had not arrived half an hour
earlier; even he could not have become impatient during the
seven minutes in which time our daughter entered the world.

Sister breezed briskly into the ward the next morning.

'So you have your little girl again,' she said, placing her into
my arms; I smiled contentedly; it was too early for ecstasy; contentment was all that I could manage.

Despite trying to remain on an emotionally even keel, I
nevertheless experienced several 'downs' during the next few
days.

The first was brought about simply by a nurse talking about
Amanda. I had tried studiously to avoid bringing the matter
up—the sudden death of a baby is not a subject to be discussed
at length in a maternity home, and I thought it was tactless and
unkind to introduce the subject in front of another mother. As
far as I was concerned, it brought the death of Amanda ines-
capably into my mind, when I had tried to leave it behind for the
moment. When my neighbour left— for she only stayed forty-
eight hours—I was left alone in the room for a night, and fears
for my new baby enveloped me. I was ill at ease, and had difficulty getting to sleep. But in the morning, all was well and my
daughter joined me once again.

A new mother then arrived, a plump Cockney girl, at twen-
ty-one, about to produce her second child. She had rather a

noisy labour, but within minutes of the birth had recovered her equilibrium and was practically bouncing with joy at the birth of a son. I couldn't help being amused at the sudden change in her, and rather wistfully compared my own exhausted state the previous day with her ebullience.

This then, I thought, is the difference that ten years makes.

I had toyed with the idea of giving the baby a name very similar to Amanda—Amy, Amabel, Annabel and so on; but in the end I gave her a completely different first name; Karen. It seemed right that a new personality should have its own name—its own separate identity. I had searched her round face for dimples like Amanda's and found none at all, and I was strangely glad; this was a new child, my third child, not a reincarnation of my second. But there was no reason why she should not bear her sister's name in addition to her own—Karen Amanda had a nice flowing sound, and the time would come when I would wish to explain the reason to her.

Several of the relations accidently called her Amanda in the next few weeks, but I was never hurt by that; two of the most hurtful remarks I experienced were actually made in the first week in the maternity home by a doctor and by a midwife.

The doctor, temporarily in charge of me, but hardly knowing me, obviously felt that some pleasantry was called for at the end of his examination of the baby. Glancing down at my case notes, he said casually, 'And will we see you back here next year?'

I was so shaken and angered by his question, that I could hardly speak, succeeding only in replying through gritted teeth, 'I sincerely hope not.'

To me his question had implied one thing—that something might happen to this baby, and although I am sure he meant no such thing, and with the passing of months and years, the offence seems trivial, it overshadowed me then for hours. No doubt in glancing down, he had seen the years set out—1967; 1969; 1970; 1971 and now 1972. He had assumed I had borne a child in each of those years, and would probably go on to produce more in subsequent years. It was not a difficult mistake to make; but I couldn't forgive him. He should have read the notes properly.

I was even more outraged by the midwife—the very midwife who had delivered small Amanda. For her remarks were made with the full knowledge of my case history.

By this time I was up and about and conversing with the midwife and one or two other girls. Turning to me she said, 'Mrs Luben, you've had two miscarriages in 1969 and 1970 and a pregnancy last year; don't you think it's about time you thought about birth control?'

I was so flabbergasted that once again, I could barely stammer out my answer.

'But you know I only became pregnant this time because of Amanda...'

I didn't know whether to be angry or insulted. Not one of my five pregnancies had been accidental. I had spent the last three years desperately trying to achieve a second child. I thought she must be quite stupid if she couldn't see that.

She went on to extol the virtues of the 'coil' which she herself had had fitted. It seemed her question had been nothing more than an introduction leading up to a sales chat about the coil and perhaps an opportunity to mention her continuing sex life in a group of much younger women. I lost a great deal of my previous respect for her. She was an excellent midwife, but as a human being she had gone down in my estimation, using such a sensitive area of my life as a stepping stone to an expression of her views.

There is no doubt, of course, that I was excessively— perhaps even obsessively—sensitive and twice I was thrown into a panic by the most trivial of events.

A few days after her birth, I was told by a nurse that Karen was to be put on three-hourly feeds, and immediately I became terrified that something was wrong with her—that she was showing signs of some frailty. I was told just before the morning rest period and I succeeded in calming myself and going off to sleep. When I awoke, I was refreshed and able to see things in perspective once again. Karen just happened to be a baby that wanted an extra feed. Indeed, the new schedule transformed her from a cross-patch to a contented baby. In retrospect, I was able to look at the flexibility shown at the maternity home with a great deal of approval. It contrasted markedly with stories of regimentation and lack of individual attention (and to their shame, discouragement of breast-feeding) I had heard about many larger hospitals.

Despite her improved temper, Karen never became a placid, sleepy baby like Robert. I was surprised to find that even in the ten day stint in the maternity home, she was amazingly wide awake, staring out from her cot with blue eyes.

Matron came in one morning with the post and glancing down at her, asked, 'Was your baby premature?'

'No,' I replied. 'She was full term—why?'

'Oh, she has "prem eyes".'

I stared at Karen's eyes—slightly slanted at the corners—was there something I had missed—something wrong that was only just being noticed? For several feeds, I could hardly bear to hold her—I was so sure that something was wrong. Then sanity returned; she was a lovely and perfect child; bright and alert. There was nothing wrong with her. The fault was in me.

Towards the end of my stay, I was allowed to start changing nappies.

'Isn't this a day early?' I asked my Indian nurse, remembering the routine from the earlier occasions.

'Sister sees you are a good mother,' she replied, smiling. 'She knows you can cope with the baby.'

'Oh, I don't think that's got anything to do with it,' I laughed, but I was pleased at the suggestion that it could be so.

In fact many of the experienced mothers were allowed to take over the care of their babies earlier than usual. The home was particularly busy, with a regular flow of incoming women, and two or three babies were being born every day. Once again, I was impressed that the usual routine was able to be changed, rather than rigidly adhered to, so that nurses were freed from nappy changing and baby bathing to attend at deliveries and assist new mothers.

Sister was a disciplinarian—she had to be—but she knew when to slacken the reins, and when to change the rules. Once I saw her speedily making up a bed during a rush and my admiration for her increased. She was ready to step into any gap to keep this place running smoothly.

The day before I was due to leave, she approached me.

'I shan't be here tomorrow, as it's my day off, so I'll say "goodbye" now.'

We shook hands and I was aware of a feeling of a mutual unexpressed respect that had not been present before. Perhaps we had each learned to look beneath the surface.

One Day at a Time

My mother was disappointed when I said we wouldn't go to Brighton on my departure from the maternity home. She thought perhaps that last summer's pleasant days might be repeated—but I was not tempted. I wanted no carbon copy of the previous year. Life is like a moving staircase— life had, thank goodness, moved on for me. I had no wish to stop it and make some sentimental journey back to past days.

In any case, whilst the circumstances looked the same on the surface—another daughter, another summer—things were changing drastically. In just over a week, Robert would start school—I felt a great need for stabilising— for getting into some sort of routine before school imposed its own much more demanding routine upon me.

A nearish neighbour, whose daughter had befriended Robert during the past couple of years, had kindly volunteered to take him to the school bus stopping point each morning, at what was a hectic time for me; it was some weeks before I found that Karen was sleeping until around nine a.m., and I could slip out myself with Robert just before eight-thirty to deliver him to the bus stop. He needed this little support from me; he made no complaint about school, except to comment in a weary little voice: 'It's a very tiring day.'

I was well aware that he had been flung in at the deep end, to sink or swim as best he could, in the school adventure, whilst the emotional impact on me of seeing my first born depart for school was greatly muted by having a new baby to care for. We were often irritable with each other, both exhausted by our different efforts; violent arguments were frequent and always bitterly regretted later. Poor Robert, he had borne the brunt of all the dips and peaks of my emotions, through four pregnancies and three disappointments. Somehow he had remained sufficiently well balanced to deal with the new trauma of school in a remarkably stoical fashion. He never wept on departing for school, yet he was a lonely and shy little boy and it must have been an ordeal for him to be confronted with so many noisy children in those first few months, having been a lone wolf for so many years.

Once he sat on a stool by the side of Karen's cot and I heard him say, 'Now Karen, I'm going to tell you all about an engine.'

He had needed a companion for so long. Was it too late now, I wondered? Was the gap between them permanently unbridgeable?

At least pint-sized Karen had some function—merely putting her pram in the garden gave him the confidence to play out there, for he had not lost his fear of being alone in the apparently vast open space.

Very soon after her birth he asked me, 'Will this baby die too, Mummy?'

I could only answer in the way I had answered myself: 'I don't think God would be so unkind as to take this baby from us.'

But who could be sure? If there was no God then nothing was sure; I had to turn myself away from that line of reasoning.

'Oh, God,' I would say. 'You have tried my strength; I have tried to be strong, but please don't ask me to go through it again. Please don't let anything happen to this baby. I don't think I could survive it.'

In the middle of September, the New Year edition of the Synagogue Newsletter arrived at our house. Quickly I leafed through it, and then felt a surge of excitement as I discovered my own article faithfully reproduced in its entirety.

Once again, I experienced a tremendous elation that was related as much to seeing my own name at the head of the article as to my success in publicising the nature of 'cot death'.

Within a week or so, I sent the article to my contact, Dr Knight, at the British Guild, anxious to receive praise for my efforts. But, in spite of receiving welcome words of encouragement, I had to forego any further writing for the time being.

Later the desire to write was to bubble up, reminding me of

its existence, refusing to be pushed aside again. Words, descriptions would form in my mind, as I worked around the house, but for the moment there was no room in the already tight schedule for any extras.

The most restful part of each day was the time I spent feeding Karen; blissfully I would sink on to my bed with my feet up, putting baby to the breast. How I appreciated those precious, peaceful moments. Once I had said, 'A new baby is nothing more than a parasite, taking all and giving nothing. It's constantly making demands—feeding, changing, bathing and so on—and complains when it doesn't get what it wants.'

Now, I reflected on how relaxing it was to deal with a baby after a demanding five year old. It didn't argue, shout, fight, ask questions or make silly jokes. All it required was to be clean and fed and it was contented. How the perspective had changed.

Karen was only five weeks old when we visited Michael's mother on a pleasant October Sunday. Karla, my sister-in-law, who had a cold, telephoned to ask my feelings about her being there. It may have seemed excessively protective, but I had to say that I couldn't deliberately allow Karen to be exposed to an infection, however mild, at that age. So Karla nobly stayed at home while the rest of us enjoyed a family occasion. I had brought my camera and we photographed the six cousins together—eleven year old Stephen holding the baby and the other little boys arranged sitting and standing around. Then I held Karen while Michael photographed the two of us—at my request. Amanda's photographs had meant a great deal to me, and I wanted to be sure I had a record of Karen.

I lived with fear, but I accepted its presence as inevitable. The possibility of losing Karen could not be put from my mind, unlikely though it may have seemed to anyone else; now, as we entered the time of year when respiratory ailments were more common, I was aware of her increased vulnerability.

One morning, I spent five or ten minutes chatting with the other mothers at the bus-stop. As I left them, I was overcome with guilt at having left Karen unattended for such a long time. I ran panting back to the house, petrified at what I might find.

The terrible panics occurred often, and each time, weak with relief, I would find a contented sleeping baby in the cot.

Autumn crept past. Robert had mumps—and two bouts of bronchitis—but Karen was not affected.

Twice I myself went to the doctor with the first symptoms of a cold.

'Is there anything,' I asked, 'that can stop it in its tracks?'

The doctor gave me something, and the cold did not develop. Goodness knows if it was psychological, for there is no cure, as we all know, for the common cold. But the desired result was achieved; baby Karen did not catch a cold from me or anyone else during her first winter.

Sometimes I would hold her in my arms, and gaze at her thinking, 'If you were to die tomorrow, I would have had this moment.'

Each night I had to discipline myself to go to sleep; there would be no advantage to any member of the family, if I lay awake night after night in fear. So I would check her, listen to the quiet breathing, see the pink tones of her skin in the half light, and then walk out of the door. In my own bedroom, I would turn up the newly acquired baby alarm, listen again to the sound of even breathing, and then turn it right down, so that I could only hear her if she cried.

Once or twice my nerve failed, and I would rush to her cot again. Sometimes a gentle touch to her body would immediately awaken her, for she was an extremely light sleeper, and I would have to give her a late night feed. Michael would grumble, 'Have you woken her up again?' He didn't have my personality—he didn't know of my fears—luckily for both of us. And when in the middle of the night, cries of hunger or thirst would shrill out, instead of blearily cursing, I always opened my eyes and thought, 'Thank God, she's alive.'

But it was not an unhappy time—far from it. The insecurity lent a special value to her babyhood; each day was a heaven sent gift. I was aware now that I had allowed Robert's baby days to fly past unappreciated, always watching impatiently for the next stage. Now as precious moments were savoured, I realised that I had actually gained something from Amanda's death. For these days poised between terror and ecstasy had a bitter-sweet quality, and with the contrast of black days behind me, normality had suddenly become technicolour.

I could remember with clarity that a year ago, I thought no-one else had ever suffered such a blow. To lose husband, wife, brother or sister could not be so bad as to lose one's baby, I had secretly told myself. Humbly now, I recognised the arrogance of that assumption.

On the contrary, I now felt privileged to have suffered the year of bereavement, without which I would not have known this magical contrast.

In addition, Amanda's death had not been a totally meaningless event as I had once bitterly thought, for it had caused me to grow up and look beyond my own needs, to see if I could help other people.

Amanda, who had no life of her own, would nevertheless be remembered through anything I could do on her behalf.

Spring came and passed, with its progress marked by the appearance of each new wave of flowers—the early bulbs, polyanthus, wallflowers, my own daffodils, and the many coloured tulips. At the end of April, Karen was eight months old. It was a milestone—the period of greatest risk of cot death is between two and eight months, the most dangerous time of year, between October and April. But still, another month passed before I felt entirely safe.

Then suddenly it was June. Suddenly the sun was shining down. In a spontaneous expression of joy, I ran outside and across the garden. The air was warm, the sky blue and the green grass firm and springy beneath my feet. I felt a moment's solid happiness, tempered then, momentarily by a swift fear. Nothing is ever sure; at each new stage of my baby's life, there would be new dangers.

But at least she would not slip away in the night without warning. She was mine now, really mine. And in that moment of happiness, I remembered again the commitment I had made.

For a while, in a period of almost religious ecstasy, I believed

I had found the answer to the tribulations of the world. God, I thought, did not necessarily spare us from all grief, but He did give us a remarkable ability to survive it, and the extraordinary happiness after the period of extreme pain was surely an enormous compensation for that pain.

But later humility followed. I could not, after all, justify the hideous suffering in the world; I could only see a purpose in my own period of sorrow.

There came a time when I became complacent about my experience of bereavement and felt almost impatient with mothers who did not seem to be making a recovery from the death of a baby. Then I realised that I was making the same mistake that others had made and which had upset me at the time. No doubt they had said, 'She's young; she'll have another baby; she'll get over it.' But it is simply not possible for a mother to look at the death of her baby in the long term. However good is the eventual prognosis of her recovery, it does not heal the sharp pain of the moment.

In the five years following Karen's birth, I wrote to several women whose names were passed to me. Sometimes the correspondence lasted for months with the exchange of seven or eight letters, each one, for me, an outpouring of past emotions. I also succeeded in getting letters and articles on cot death published in newspapers and magazines.

In 1975, I felt sufficiently detached from the situation to hold a coffee morning to raise funds for the Foundation, and this has become a small annual practice. On one of those occasions, I met a mother who, until that day, had been unable to accept the death of her baby, but at least after that, was able to express her feelings of sorrow.

I am aware that numerically my efforts seem trivial, but at least they have been consistent, and when at any time I have been made aware of a mother grieving for a lost baby, my response has been immediate.

Although, as a result of fund-raising, much useful research has been and continues to be carried out, the precise cause of cot death remains unexplained. It is suggested that S.I.D.S.

probably results not from a single cause but from a variety of different factors which combine fatally while a child is passing through a vulnerable period of development

But parents suddenly bereaved are much more likely now to receive automatic support, as a result of the work done by the Foundation and the British Guild, than they would have been at the time of Amanda's death and before, and in this respect, real progress has been made.

My children are no longer babies; to describe their lives and personalities now would be unfair to two young people who have not sought the limelight. Suffice it to say that Robert's confidence increased and he became totally at home in the once alien woods and amongst his own group of friends. As Karen grew older, they grew together and were, after all, companions in games and squabbles and many other interests. Both children, with all their imperfections, seem very satisfactory to me.

In the garden, my spindly fuchsia survived for many years, flowering briefly each year from early August to the first frost. When weather or disease or some other pest destroyed it, I did not replace it. We lost the plum trees, the pear trees and three of the apple trees. But the last apple eventually produced many crops and by then I had learned to be philosophical. Just as I waited for my unborn children and was eventually thankful and grateful for what I received, so I accepted in the same spirit, the harvest of fruit from the trees.

Useful Addresses

COT DEATH

Foundation for the Study of Infant Deaths
(Cot Death Research and Support)
Artillery House,
11-19 Artillery Row,
London, SW1P 1RT.
Helpline: 020 7233 2090

Irish SIDS Association
Carmichael House,
4, North Brunswick Street,
Dublin 7.
Helpline: 1850 391391

Scottish Cot Death Trust
Royal Hospital for Sick Children,
Yorkhill,
Glasgow, G3 8SJ.
Helpline: 0141 357 3946

MISCARRIAGE and STILLBIRTH

Miscarriage Association
c/o Clayton Hospital, Northgate,
Wakefield, W. Yorkshire, WF1 3JS.
Helpline: 01924 200799
Scottish Helpline (Answerphone): 0131 334 8883

Stillbirth and Neonatal Death Society (SANDS)
28, Portland Place,
London, W1N 4DE.
Helpline: 020 7436 5881

BEREAVEMENT AND GENERAL

Compassionate Friends
53, North Street,
Bedminster,
Bristol, BS3 1EN
Helpline: 0117 953 9639

Cruse - Bereavement Care
126, Sheen Road,
Richmond,
Surrey, TW9 1UR.
Helpline: 0208 332 7277

National Childbirth Trust (NCT)
Alexandra House,
Oldham Terrace,
Acton,
London, W3 6NH.
Tel: 020 8992 8637

Tamba (Twins and Multiple Births Association)
Harnott House,
309, Chester Road,
Little Sutton,
Ellesmere Port, CH66 1QQ.
Tel: 0870 121 4000